CHRIS IMBO'S PEAK 10 FITNESS

"The Best of New York . . . Best Personal Trainer—Chris Imbo."
—New York

"Peak 10 . . . whips you into the best shape genetics and willpower will allow."
—Allure

"I was amazed by the results I saw in only one week, and I believed more and more in Peak 10 every week."
—ELLE

Chris Imbo, the ACSM and ACE certified trainer, is also owner and director of CASA, a specialized private fitness club in New York City. His three-pronged approach to total fitness is based on *exercise* to burn fat, boost metabolism and carve muscles, combined with *nutrition* and *attitude* to deliver lasting results!

CHRIS △ IMBO'S PEAK ⟵→ 10. FITNESS

CHRIS AND SALLY IMBO

with Donna Raskin

A PERIGEE BOOK

A Perigee Book
Published by The Berkley Publishing Group
200 Madison Avenue
New York, NY 10016

First edition: March 1996

Published simultaneously in Canada.

The Putnam Berkley World Wide Web site address is http://www.berkley.com

Library of Congress Cataloging-in-Publication Data

Imbo, Chris.
    [Peak 10 fitness]
    Chris Imbo's peak 10 fitness / Chris and Sally Imbo with Donna
Raskin.—1st ed.
        p.   cm.
    "A Perigee book."
    ISBN 0-399-51984-X
    1. Physical fitness.   2. Exercise.   I. Imbo, Sally.   II. Raskin,
Donna.   III. Title.   IV. Title: Peak 10 fitness
GV481.I53   1996
613.7'1—dc20   95-38210
                                                         CIP

Printed in the United States of America

10   9   8   7   6   5   4   3   2   1

To my wife, Sally Belle

Contents

Acknowledgments

Many people have helped me put together this book. I would like to thank everyone who has been so supportive. From the beginning, Martha McCully has been there as a sounding board for my ideas, helping me discover new ways to keep people interested in fitness. Joel Lulla, besides his entertainment qualities, has been instrumental in the formation of Imbo International, Inc., and all of the projects that I've been involved in.

Thanks to Julie Merberg for being such a pleasure to work with, for her patience, and for pulling an all-nighter to complete this before deadline. Donna Raskin kept pace after moving across the country; thanks for sticking to it, Donna.

Thank you to my trainers for working such long hours and for trusting in me. Thank you to all my "Peakies," for giving it their all. Thanks to Mark Terk for his friendship and expert photography and for knowing his way around a menu. Thank you to Stu Mittleman, who taught me so much about exercise physiology and has been a great friend and comrade.

Many thanks to my family and friends, especially my wonderful son T. Rex, and of course, thanks to Sally for being my perfect complement.

—Chris Imbo

I would like to thank Chris for thinking of me and also for being a very motivational trainer. He has changed my life and the way I think about my body. I would also like to thank Julie Merberg for being perhaps the most patient editor on earth. Then there's Deborah Kasdan, who helped me mature as a writer and editor. My friends Kate, Kathy, Madonna, and Dana are gifts from God and I thank him for them every day. Also my friends Steve, Susan, Stephani and Nick, who are gifts from earth, which oddly enough makes them particularly inspirational. Finally, I would like to thank my mother, my father, and my stepfather, as well as my brothers and sisters, because my family is supportive and encouraging all the time and in their own special way.

—Donna Raskin

1

Welcome to Peak 10

Being fit, lean, and healthier are all within your power. I honestly believe that attaining the body and fitness you desire takes only small modifications in your everyday life, and those alterations begin with three things: knowledge, commitment, and guidance.

You're about to become a member of a very exclusive group of people who have already used Peak 10 to achieve their fitness and health goals. The Peak 10 program is not just another "get fit quick" program. It is the reality check we've all needed for a long time. You must believe that there are no magic pills, no secret potions, or anything other than your own desire and belief in the true fundamentals of fitness that will change you. With my support and guidance you will finally take charge of the way you look and feel.

Peak 10, a ten-week program I developed over the course of 5 years, is the practical integration of the most sensible eating and exercise knowledge wrapped up in one program. It doesn't matter what shape you are in now or how much fat you think you need to lose: Together we will attain your goals.

My goal—and the goal of Peak 10—is to create a way of life that gives you an optimum level of energy, fitness, and health. By following this program daily for ten weeks, you will develop the habits that make regular exercise and a good diet the norm, and not something you wish you could squeeze into your already crazy schedule.

No matter what point you're at when you start, you have to know exactly where you want to wind up. Do you want to be leaner? More toned? Have a flatter stomach? Thinner thighs? Do you want to run a marathon? Play a set of singles without getting tired? The choices are yours. Then we have to create a plan to get you what you want. We're going to do it together, taking stock of what we have and what we need. We will redesign your body's blueprint so that you will be the best that genetics will allow. After ten weeks you won't simply be at the end of a journey, you will be at the beginning of a whole new life.

This doesn't mean you won't see changes or get results right away. You'll definitely notice a difference after the first two weeks, I promise.

By focusing on your health and fitness for just ten weeks, you'll learn new behaviors that will become second nature—enabling you to become your physical best. In general, Peak 10 involves learning how to incorporate a convenient, low-fat, highly nutritious eating plan with exercise. We determine your personal aerobic training zone so you can burn body fat, and then we'll also add a strength training program to increase muscle tone and boost your metabolism. Adding all of these elements to your life will bring about swift changes to your body and your state of mind. My clients—people of all ages, shapes, sizes, and fitness levels—have lost fat and strengthened their bodies, thereby increasing lean muscle mass. They have reconditioned their bodies to burn fat, not store it. The more lean muscle mass you have, the more calories and fat your body will burn at work and at rest. The program has worked for others, and it will work for you too.

IT'S SIMPLE

It might sound funny, but even though Peak 10 isn't easy, it's simple. Each step taken on its own builds on the one that came before. Each day of the program will be structured for you to follow. And when you look back at the whole ten weeks, you'll realize that it wasn't a lot of time to dedicate to one of your most important assets. But, as I said, simple doesn't mean easy. You will have to make a commitment to work with me and dig deep inside yourself to find the strength to keep pushing. You have to push through the years of what I call negative conditioning, the patterns you have learned and practiced your entire life that leave you still struggling.

I've seen people succeed and I've seen people struggle. I know that this program is challenging, but I can help you through it. All it takes is a dedicated effort fused with enthusiastic support and guidance from me. We will monitor and evaluate your progress as we move forward. Together, we will recondition your mind and body for a lifetime of peak health.

The objective of Peak 10 is to get results as quickly and safely as possible. And nothing will motivate you more than seeing your body change right before your eyes. As your fat level decreases, you might notice that your clothes fit better. You might have to tighten your belt a notch or two, or perhaps that jacket that used to fit looks great on you again. Maybe a friend or family member will notice the change in the way you look and carry yourself. These progressive changes will give you the inspiration to stick with the program. Every day of success will lead you into another day of more success.

For me, fitness means being in control of how I look and feel twenty-four hours a day. Fitness means being able to go through life from the moment you wake up to the moment you go to bed in a state of balance—coping with being stressed-out, anxious, or run-down. Fitness is looking your best, being the best, feeling healthy and strong. And it can happen without having to crash-diet or exercise until you're exhausted or blue in the face (which is a real no-no). Being fit must simply be part of your life.

TAKE SOME TIME

Most of my clients are busy, high-powered individuals. Their time is both valuable and limited, just like yours. There are only so many hours in a day. My clients—and perhaps you—think it's difficult to make room for fitness, but if you *live* fitness, and I mean really understand what it takes to be healthy and fit, it becomes automatic. A fit life is one in which a natural amount of exercise and healthful eating work together to maintain your fitness. It's not necessarily about having a gym membership or a stair machine in your bedroom (we all know cardio equipment can be a great place to hang your clothes). It's about having the knowledge and understanding of what it takes to be your best. You can't "Just Do It" if you don't know what to do!

Yes, the Peak 10 program requires a major commitment to instigate change; but once you've completed the program, a minimal time commitment will be enough for you to maintain and continue to improve your new body.

GET TO KNOW YOUR BODY

In the beginning you have to take some time to learn about your body. You must learn what your body requires in order to exist in a healthy state at all times. What foods make you feel good (and don't make you fat)? Which exercises give you more energy and keep your body strong? Which muscles are in relatively good shape? And which ones feel like they've never been used before? With your commitment, it will take ten weeks to learn these things and get used to the changes, but after that, the knowledge is yours forever. The transformation will take place and fitness will be less time-consuming. Fitness will become a foundation for everything you do.

People go to school to learn a trade, then they go on to take a job and apply the information they've learned. That's just what you're going to do: This is an education in fitness, and you're about to learn how to go forward and live a healthy life.

Of the hundreds of people I've worked with, I've never met *anyone* who didn't have room for physical improvement, and that includes celebrities, models, and athletes. The most exciting thing for me is to see someone really succeed. I've worked with some clients who started out barely able to walk at a slow pace for twenty minutes, and by the end of ten weeks they were able to jog comfortably for more than a half hour. That's not even the most exciting part. What's really thrilling is to see them out running *by themselves* three months later.

Like you, I have control over one true thing in my life, and that's my body. Sure, I'll never be six feet tall and I'll say good-bye to more and more hair every morning until they perfect a cure for baldness. I've got to work with what I have, just as everyone does. But fortunately, we each control what we put in our mouths and how active a life we will lead. Let's find out what you have to work with and take control of what you want for yourself.

"I had one chance in life and I wasn't the best I could be," says one of my clients, Carol Lynde, who reduced her percentage of body fat from 41 to 26 in ten weeks. "I wasn't taking care of myself and I needed to learn how. It's the one thing I can control, it's the one thing that isn't influenced by outside forces."

BE IN CONTROL

Understanding what you have control over and being at your physical best will eliminate a lot of fear in other areas of your life. The sensation of being in control—feeling comfortable with mastery—will overflow into other things you do. I believe that if you tackle the situation where you have the most control—your fitness—then situations where you have less control will seem less intimidating. The basic principles of Peak 10— *establishing where you are, determining where you want to go, and defining how you will get there*—can be applied to nearly any task you wish to conquer.

Since the best results in life come when you have a good teacher who listens to your goals and helps you create a program to achieve them, it was smart of you to look for a coach. As your coach, I won't just teach you to "listen to your body," I'll teach you to process information from your body. We'll create two open lines of communication, one between you and your body, and one between you and me.

WHAT'S IT LIKE?

"I loved the whole process of Peak 10," says Martha McCully, a magazine editor. "The plunge into self-absorption helped me redefine myself, and not just physically. For ten weeks, Peak 10 became my priority." Martha started the program at 29 percent body fat and ended it at 17 percent. She lost nineteen pounds of body fat. Her exercise schedule included working out with weights in the morning and doing a walk/run in the afternoons.

"I look back at Peak 10 as a real emotional experience—a defining moment—of my life," Martha continues. "Today I maintain a better body than I ever had, and I still exercise three times a week."

Today, after years of dieting prior to doing Peak 10, Martha enjoys good health and a high level of fitness. "Before Peak 10 I went on a lot of traditional diets. It was always such a struggle to maintain a body that didn't feel natural to me, but now nutritionally I'm a different person. There was so much focus on myself. It made me want to succeed."

Peak 10 doesn't only work for women. One of my clients, Steve Friedman, is an editor at *GQ* magazine in New York City. "I was overwhelmed when I first moved to New York," Steve explains. "I had the flu about five times and couldn't find a basketball game or a place to swim like I had in St. Louis, so I got soft and flabby."

Steve joined a gym, but didn't know how to use the cardiovascular equipment properly, so I taught him what he needed to know to reach his goals. Steve's body fat was over 20 percent, which is high for a man. His cholesterol count was also high. It indicated that he wasn't as healthy as he could be.

After ten weeks Steve's body changed. "I had all my clothes tailored," Steve says, "and a year later I'm still wearing the smaller sizes. I've kept my body fat and cholesterol levels down." What made the difference? "I'd never used weights before, and learning about their effectiveness was incredible. Chris is after results, but he's not obsessed. He's after balance."

I *am* after balance. In fact, let me tell you a little about myself and the evolution of Peak 10.

HOW I DEVELOPED PEAK 10

I haven't always led a balanced lifestyle. Before I became a trainer I worked on Wall Street and pushed myself to my limits both physically and mentally. Working long hours and living a lifestyle of fast food and after-dinner drinks was self-destructive for me. I allowed myself to get caught up in a pattern of bad habits that proved nearly impossible to break. The foods of mainstream America were pulsing through my veins and clogging my arteries. With a history of heart disease in my family, I realized that this could lead me to an early grave unless I took control. I was becoming spongy, even at the young age of twenty-four. But scariest of all, I resembled all the other guys in my age group. When I looked at the guys who were five or ten years older, I knew this life wasn't for me.

I was determined to change myself, and I did. So I understand the challenges that you're about to face. As a society we are being challenged every step of the way. For example, the way we celebrate the important events in our lives—weddings, birthdays—encourages overindulgence in food, alcohol, and all the stuff we're supposed to avoid. But while you *can* avoid fat, you *can't* avoid food, so it is very important that we adjust. Understanding balance and moderation, and practicing these ideals, will ease the wonderful metamorphosis that you'll experience before long.

As a personal trainer, I want to make sure my clients continue to use my services, and they do when they see significant results. I keep detailed records of the progress each client makes both by taking measurements and by adding new, more challenging exercises. I always ask them, "How are you doing?" "How are you feeling?" "Anything hurt?" to get as much feedback as possible. Over the years I learned a lot about what works and what doesn't when a person wants to get into shape.

One of the biggest challenges of personal training comes right at the beginning of a program. Most clients have let much time and many a donut come between them and being fit. So it becomes a game of catch-up. All of a sudden they need to get into shape in two months for some special event where they must look great. The first thing I do is to separate fact from fiction. I make my evaluation, ask all the necessary questions. Then we set our goals, but we're realistic and conservative. I make it clear that slow and gradual is the only way to go. They usually ask what they can expect, at which point I tell them what fifteen pounds of fat looks like. It's not pretty, and it's not so easy to shake it.

It's my job to get my client—in this case you—where you want to be. If you want to get into a smaller pant size in a certain amount of time, I'll get you there, but it would be irresponsible of me to get you to that special event (the class reunion, your sister's wedding, or even bathing-suit season) and not take you through the day after. With Peak 10 I'm determined to get you into shape for that momentous occasion and then take you even further. I'm going to make sure you eat right and exercise correctly for the rest of your life.

Once you're in Peak 10 condition, I guarantee that you'll maintain your fit body after the program. In fact, determining how to keep that level of fitness was partly how the program was developed.

For many, Peak 10 can be an emotional overhaul. But let's face it: Most people exercise and eat a low-fat diet because they want to *look* good. I don't think that's such a horrible thing. In fact, I believe that along the way to beauty, we've all learned a lot about health and fitness. We've learned that the underlying structure of good looks is good health. Attractiveness is about feeling good about yourself.

The Program

The most important thing I've discovered as a trainer is that you don't have to kill yourself to be in great shape. If you exercise and eat right, the balance of good health comes naturally. That's the philosophy I give to my clients.

The first step of Peak 10 is for you to understand the commitment you're making. Your life and health are wonderful gifts. I'm dedicated to helping you make the process of learning and changing as motivating, realistic, fun and effective as possible.

The second step of the program is an overall health and fitness evaluation. Together we'll find out what your body-fat percentage is, figure out what kind of shape you're in, and determine your aerobic heart rate training zone for maximum fat-loss capability.

During the third phase of the program, you'll determine what goals you want to reach at the end of Peak 10. You can only set the goals after knowing where you are now. You will want to aim for realistic, informed goals that are reachable without running yourself into the ground.

With the above information added to the knowledge that I'll pass on to you about eating right and exercising progressively, you'll create a program guaranteed to change your body.

While on Peak 10, you'll eat three meals and two or three snacks a day. Carbohydrates will make up about 70 percent of the calories you eat, protein about 15 percent, and fat about 15 percent. I'm going to make sure you get through the day with a lot of energy by eating a sufficient number of calories. However, we'll create a caloric deficit, so you'll burn body fat and boost your metabolism without being hungry or tired.

Cardiovascular conditioning will be divided into two components: one to strengthen your cardiovascular system and the other to burn fat. Both will include a warm-up, a training "core," and a cool-down.

Weight training will be done three days a week, skipping days to allow the body to rest and recover.

Throughout the program you'll get the benefit of my personal experiences backed up by guidelines from both the American College of Sports Medicine and the American Heart Association. Each week we'll check in with our numbers to see that we're moving in the right direction. Remember, ten weeks is long enough to change and modify your behavior, but not too long that you'll get bored, give up, or quit.

We often think of good health as the absence of a complaint. In fact, perhaps we think of good health as something we shouldn't have to think about. But I believe our health is more than that. Good health is a spark, a vitality, a ripeness or a richness of life. It allows us to respond to and enjoy each part of our lives. Good health, fitness, and strength are not ends in themselves; they are starting points from which we can leap into the parts of our lives we care most about: our families, our careers, our roles as friend, partner, and human being with valuable ideas and purpose. But most important, I want you to be able to enjoy and experience what life has to offer for as long as you can. It won't hurt to look great along the way.

Good health is not about excessive training or starvation diets. It is simply a balance of ourselves in nature. For each of my clients, that has meant something different. Whatever good health means to you, whatever fitness means for you, I can help you get—and stay—healthy and fit.

KRISTEN'S STORY

I did Peak 10 because I was unhappy about how I felt about myself: fat and out of shape. It wasn't about how other people viewed me. I'm a big

Kristen Age: 24 Height: 5'11"	*Start*	*Finish*
MEASUREMENTS		
Neck	13.75	13
Shoulders	41.75	40.25
Chest	40.5	38
Waist	31.5	30.5
Hips	39.75	39.5
Rt. Thigh	23.5	20.75
Rt. Calf	15	14.25
Rt. Upper Arm	11.25	10.25
Rt. Forearm	10	9.5
Weight	168 lbs.	156 lbs.
% Fat	30.6/30	22.9/23
TOTAL INCHES	227	216
Inches lost: 11		

girl and I didn't want to look husky. I wanted to do something that would make me feel better, but not kill me.

I was always thin until I went to college, then I gained thirty pounds. I would try to lose it, but only some of it would come off and the rest would stay on. I used to be a dancer, which was my primary exercise, but I found out I had a heart problem and I didn't know what I could and couldn't do. The doctor told me Peak 10 was okay, as long as I watched my heart rate, and that was part of Chris' program anyway.

It was a little tough to change the way I ate and exercised, but only for a couple of days. Chris told me something that I never forgot each time I wanted to pig out: "Every time you turn down a cookie or potato chip you're ahead of everybody and you're ahead of yourself. Every little thing counts."

The exercise I did really gave me peace of mind. I felt a lot better about myself. The weight didn't fall off right away, but I knew it would eventually—and it did. I did weights a couple of days a week and I did cardiovascular every single day. I had a dyna band and light weights at home. I discovered that I really like to powerwalk. I'd walk for an hour, but sometimes it would turn into two hours because I got addicted to it. It made me happy and I got a high from doing it.

I used to eat just when I was hungry. I'd pick up something and eat it. I thought I had a low-fat diet, but I found out from Chris that I ate a lot of high-fat foods, like hummus. Now, I'm aware. I still ask people questions about food. I eat a lot of black beans and rice. I don't eat as much bread as I used to eat. I'm big on salads. I learned to enjoy vegetables and fruit.

I lost close to 20 pounds. Everything was tighter. I lost inches. I was feeling sexier and men were noticing me. I felt more confident and it made me feel like I could accomplish more. I put on a bikini this summer and I felt so great in it. Everybody noticed.

It was nice having Chris there to hold my hand while I learned Peak 10. I've tried other programs that I would start and quit, but the way Chris interacted with me really made a difference. Still, the program's success depends on the self-discipline of the person doing it.

During the winter I put a couple of pounds back on, but they're already off because of the nice weather—I'm walking everywhere again. Chris gives you the tools to do it yourself. He taught me that I can do this myself.

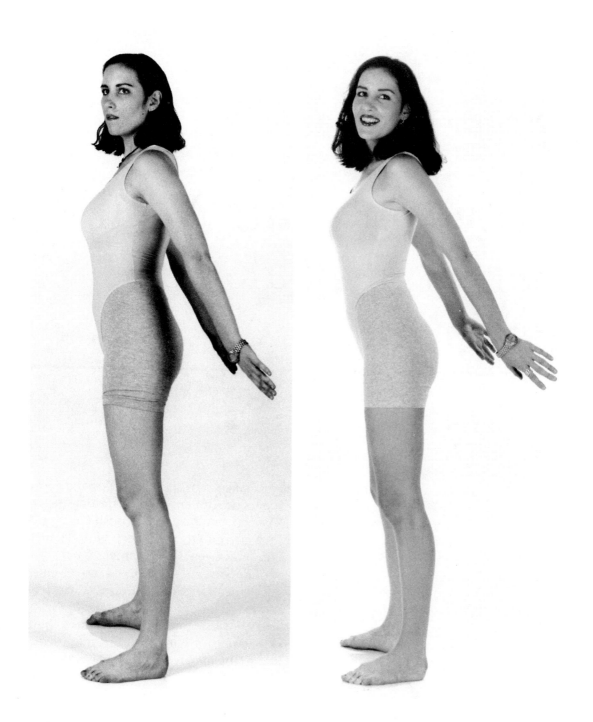

2

How to Create Your Personal Peak 10 Program

The idea of personal training is to make your body healthier and more attractive through the hands-on encouragement of your trainer. A personal trainer is someone who knows you well enough to push you a little bit further than you think you can go and who will keep very detailed records of your progress and accomplishments. He is someone who will encourage you to set and reach your goals and to help you move out of your comfort zone.

I won't be able to ring your doorbell every morning to get you out of bed for your morning aerobic work, but I'm going to try to set off some bells in your head that will make it easier for you to get up and do your thing. You as an individual will fit into the plan we've created because we all share some basic similarities. My experiences with my Peak 10 clients will empower you to move forward and be the best you can be. Now my focus is on you. I'm reaching out my hand for you to take hold of throughout the program.

When we first meet, I don't lecture clients about nutrition and exercise, I ask questions. How's your health? What are your eating habits? How often do you exercise? How do you feel about your body? What's motivated you to inquire about Peak 10? What do you want to achieve? Then, together, we plan a Peak 10 program that will get results. The more I know about my clients, the more successful they are in the program. The same is true for you. The more you know about yourself—from the basics of weight and measurements, fitness level, body-fat percentage, to your more complex needs and desires—the greater and more lasting the results you will achieve on Peak 10. We have to find out where you are now.

As I said in the first chapter, the first thing we need is knowledge. Since we learn more easily when we write information down, it's time to get out a notebook and pen or pencil. You are going to set up your own Peak 10 diary. We're going to record a lot of information throughout the ten weeks we work together.

Most people come to see me with a dream about their bodies and I'm sure you have an image, too, about your "perfect" body. So here's your chance to tell me about yourself. What do you want to look like? How do you want to feel? Do you picture yourself wearing a thong bathing suit on a Hawaiian beach or are you crossing the finish line in the New York City Marathon with a satisfied grin? Do you want to be able to keep up with your highly charged two-year-old or is there a pair of pants that you wore ten years ago that you want to fit into?

The first thing I'd like you to do is write down the image you have of *your* "perfect body." Then explain why, deep down in your heart, you are doing Peak 10. What do you most want to accomplish?

Now, in order to get to where you want to go, we have to determine where you are now. That means more preparation with paper and pen, as well as a tape measure, camera, stopwatch (or second hand), and ruler.

Remember, I said that Peak 10 isn't easy, but it *is* simple. You'll see that it takes dedication to stick to an eating plan and get up to exercise every day, but that it's simple once you have gathered all the health and fitness information we have available and apply it to yourself. I'm going to take you through step by step and help you to figure out how much of what foods to eat each day and determine how much you need to exercise and which exercises you should do. We just have to spend some time putting all of that information together to make sure you have a lifelong plan for a lean body and good health. After all, this plan is not intended to be just a quick fix. I'm planning on teaching you to live a healthier lifestyle from this moment forward, forever.

WHERE ARE YOU NOW?

Most of my clients have had enough of being unhappy with their bodies. They're self-conscious, but at the same time, they're willing to be weighed, poked, and prodded to reach their goal. And that's step one of Peak 10: figuring out where you are now.

Once you take stock of yourself and know your weaknesses and strengths, you'll have a much better chance of succeeding in your plan. You'll need to figure out how what you eat and drink affects your body so that you can continue to make improvements by adjusting your behavior. Instead of a declining shape as you age, yours can actually get *better* each year! You'll know which behaviors and choices got you to where you want to be.

Remember, though, that wherever you are now, whatever weight you are, however strong you are, is perfectly fine. I care for my clients just as much in the beginning as I do in the end. I appreciate and respect them— and you—right now, because you're someone who cares about your health. You're a visionary and a hard worker, two things I always admire. Even though Peak 10 will make you look better, feel better, and think toward the future, right now your focus should be completely on the present.

If you're a little afraid of finding out how much you really weigh or you're hesitant about recording the food you eat every day, remember that it's just something you need to see in order to go forward. You're not competing against anyone except your future self. We're using these numbers to chart your progress. It's a true test in the sense that your "score" is an indication of how far we need to go.

So let's really focus on where you are right now. This will be the information you build your dreams on.

The Dietary Recall

I'll let you in on a secret at the outset: We're not going to pick through your records to make sure you feel bad about yourself at the end. It's just that most people *don't know* what they eat. Or they aren't honest with themselves. From my experience, I've heard many people say they're following a healthful eating plan. But if they're not making progress, then the plan needs to be improved. You need to be able to recognize your pitfalls. For example, what is it that causes a binge?

For that reason, I want you to complete the Dietary Recall form on page 238. Following is a sample of the form so you'll know what you'll need to do. You can also copy the form into your notebook if you'd like. Despite the name "Recall," I don't want you to think back over the past week and try to recall what you ate. Instead, take the Dietary Recall with you wherever you go and write down what you eat and drink *as you eat it*. Those pages should begin to look like hell toward the end of the week, or you're not following directions. Don't be afraid of it. It should accompany you everywhere!

You need to get a good overview of the way you eat and break it down to see where your calories are coming from. We need to be sure that your food intake is balanced according to the Daily Recommended Allowances. You should be getting at least 70 percent of your calories from carbohydrates, 15 percent from protein, and about 15 percent from fat. We will help you to decipher all the charts and numbers so that you can really see where you stand.

Write everything down. Be specific. Include what you're drinking, how much of each food you're consuming, and how you're feeling when you're eating. Remember, this isn't a test, it's a log. We'll discuss what it means at the end of chapter 7 when we put together your personal Peak 10 plan.

Here's another tip: Do the Dietary Recall while you read this book, then go back and start the program. By the end of your reading, you'll have all the information you'll need to design your plan during the week that you monitor your food intake, and you will have completed the first step of Peak 10.

DIETARY RECALL

Day 1	Breakfast	Mid-morning	Lunch	Mid-afternoon	Dinner	PM Snack
Time						
Food/ Beverage						
Where are you?						
Who is with you?						
What are you doing?						
How do you feel?						

Notes:

TAKING BEFORE (AND AFTER) PHOTOGRAPHS

It's time to take your "before" pictures. Guess what most of my clients wear for this step? That's right—big T-shirts and shorts. People have a hard time because they're uncomfortable with the way they look and they can't visualize change. They're afraid to look at themselves in the mirror and they're afraid to let other people see them.

You might want to recruit a buddy to help you with this part—it just takes a couple of minutes. Ask someone you are close to and really trust. Remember, the pictures (and negatives) belong to you. You can keep them in your Peak 10 book or under your mattress if you want—just keep them. The good news is that in ten weeks when we take another set of pictures, you'll be able to see very clearly all the progress that you've made and how your body has improved.

Very often, when we look in the mirror, our eyes go straight to the part of our body we're most self-conscious of. Some of us only see our thighs or our stomach. When we focus on that one spot, we don't see it honestly anymore. It can grow or shrink depending on our mood (and what we're wearing). The goal here is to take an honest look at your picture. I won't compare you to anyone else. I want you to see yourself as you are right now so that you can appreciate the difference you'll see in just a few weeks.

So, take a deep breath. Wear light and tight clothing (as little as possible) and stand in front of a contrasting background. You might think you look better in dark colors, but you'll need the contrast to see your body. (You'll be grateful at the end of Peak 10 because you'll be able to see the changes in glorious detail.)

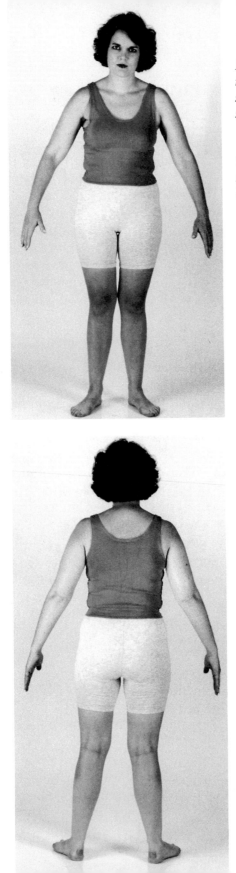

Face forward with your arms out to the side, not too far away from your body. Drop your shoulders and relax. Try not to tense up your shoulders; your body will look better relaxed.

Turn to the right and bring your arms straight back behind you, away from your body. Drop your shoulders and relax.

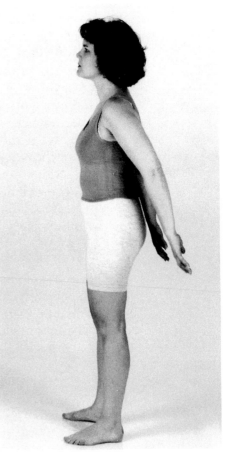

With your back to the camera, hold your arms out to the side, not too far away from your body. Once again, drop your shoulders and relax.

TAKING MEASUREMENTS

Most people get on the scale, don't like the number they see, and decide they want to lose weight. But a scale only measures how much you weigh, not what that weight is made up of. What needs to be determined is your percentage of fat-to-lean muscle mass. Two people of the same height, for example, can weigh the same amount, but one can be lean and trim while the other is flabby. What we need to know is how much excess fat is on your body. We don't want to just lose weight; we want to lose fat and inches. So we have to do more than jump on the scale and shout, "I need to lose ten pounds!" We have to say, "I have too much fat on my body and I want to gain muscle and lose the fat."

This means we have to determine your body composition. What is the ratio of fat to muscle on your body? The numbers we write down will be very important.

You'll take your measurements at nine sites on your body. Then you'll use your hip or waist measurement (depending on your gender) in ratio to your weight or height to determine your body fat. You'll also use your measurements as a baseline to chart your progress throughout Peak 10. And yes, you will weigh yourself, but please rely more on your body-fat percentage to measure your progress. It's a much more reliable indicator of your fitness level. You're going to take new measurements every two weeks.

If you're taking your own measurements, be sure not to pull too tightly on the measuring tape and don't suck in. Look in a mirror to make sure that the tape isn't drooping in the back. Write down each measurement to the nearest quarter inch on the chart on page 21. It sometimes helps to put cellophane tape on the tape measure and tape it to your body (especially when you're doing the arm measurements) in order to hold it down. You might also wrap the tape around you, match the end up, and take the tape off before reading the measurement. That sometimes makes it easier, too.

If you're worried that you're not doing it right, go through your whole body twice, then take the average of the two numbers for each site.

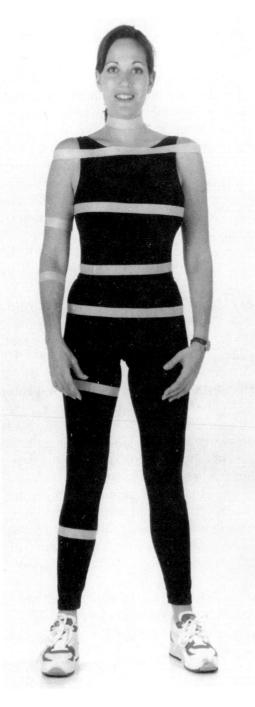

NECK: Place the tape midway between your head and shoulders.

SHOULDER: Measure your shoulders one inch below the top of your torso.

CHEST: Place the tape around your body at the nipple line.

WAIST: Measure approximately one inch above your belly button.

HIPS: Put the tape around the widest part of your hips.

RIGHT THIGH: Put your right leg forward a few inches and measure just below your buttocks.

RIGHT CALF: Measure at the widest part of your calf.

RIGHT UPPER ARM: Hold your arm straight out in front of you (palm facing up). Wrap the tape measure at the widest part of your upper arm.

RIGHT FOREARM: Still holding your arm out in front of you, measure the widest part of your forearm.

PEAK 10 PROGRESS CHART

Name: _____ **Age:** _____

	Before	Week 2	Week 4	Week 6	Week 8	Week 10
Date:						
Time:						
MEASUREMENTS (inches)						
Neck						
Shoulders						
Chest						
Waist						
Hips						
Rt. Thigh						
Rt. Calf						
Rt. Upper Arm						
Rt. Forearm						
TOTAL INCHES						
Weight						
%Fat						
Height						

As I said, we'll use these measurements as a baseline to chart your progress throughout Peak 10. We're also going to use the waist measurement (men) and the hip measurement (women) to figure out your body-fat percentage.

MEASURING BODY FAT

Measuring body fat is an inexact science. You should remember that whatever number we come up with has an error rate of plus or minus 3 percent, which means it's approximate, not a precise calculation. (The most exact way to measure body fat is by underwater, or hydrostatic, weighing, which would require submerging you in a tank full of water.) Most trainers use body-fat calipers, which also have an error rate of plus or minus 3 percent. With calipers, a trainer pinches and measures a skin fold at strategic points along the body.

Sometimes it's hard to really look at the numbers. You might be scared to find out just how much fat is on your body. Remember, this is the "before" number. In ten weeks you'll write down a very different, healthier, body-fat percentage.

We're going to use the charts below to determine your body fat. You should use this number only to chart your progress, not to judge yourself.

If you're a man, use the chart on the following page:

Body-Fat Percentage Chart for Men

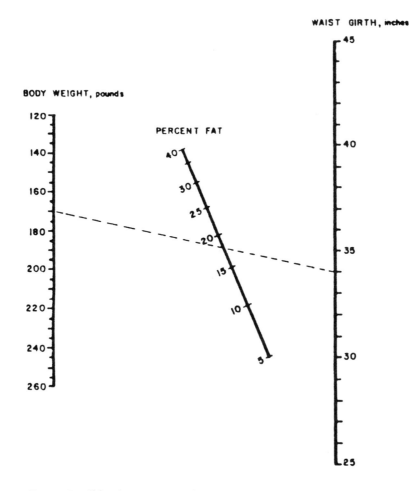

From *Sensible Fitness* (p. 30) by J.H. Wilmore, Champaign, IL: Human Kinetics Publishers. Copyright © 1986 by Jack H. Wilmore. Reprinted by permission.

Using a ruler, line up your waist measurement with your body weight. Your relative body-fat measurement is at the point where the ruler crosses the "Percent Fat" line. For example, if you're a man who weighs 170 pounds, and your waist measures 34 inches, then your body-fat percentage would be about 18. As your waist gets smaller, your body-fat percentage will lower accordingly.

If you're a woman, use this chart:

BODY-FAT PERCENTAGE CHART FOR WOMEN

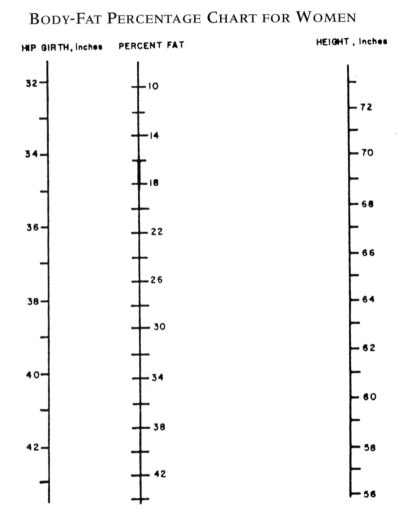

HIP GIRTH, Inches   PERCENT FAT   HEIGHT, Inches

From *Sensible Fitness* (p. 31) by J.H. Wilmore, Champaign, IL: Human Kinetics Publishers. Copyright © 1986 by Jack H. Wilmore. Reprinted by permission.

Using a ruler, line up your hip measurement with your height. Your relative body-fat measurement is at the point where the ruler crosses the "Percent Fat" line. For example, if your hips measure 36.5 inches and you are 62 inches tall (5'2"), then your body-fat percentage is about 26. Healthy levels of body fat will be discussed on page 144.

Push-up Test

Measuring Muscle Endurance

This test requires more than just measuring—you'll probably break a sweat. The best way to measure your muscular endurance is by doing a one-minute push-up test.

Now you are going to see how many push-ups you can do in one minute. Do not perform this test if you suffer from lower back ailments. There are separate procedures to be followed by males and females which are outlined below. The push-ups must be performed consecutively without a time limit, but if you can no longer keep the proper form, then you have finished the test. As with any strengthening exercise, be sure to exhale as you lift your body from the floor.

Males:

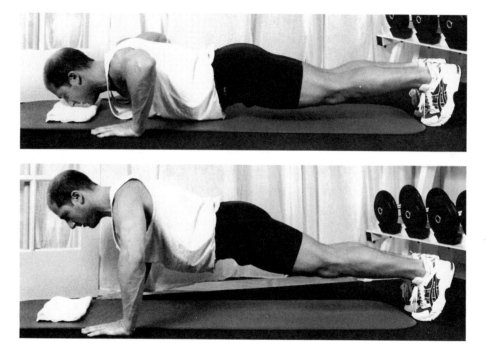

Lie on your stomach, legs together, hands pointing forward positioned under shoulders. Push up from the mat by straightening your elbows and using your toes as a pivotal point. Keep your upper body in a straight line. Return to the starting position, chin to the mat, without letting your stomach or thighs touch the mat.

Females:

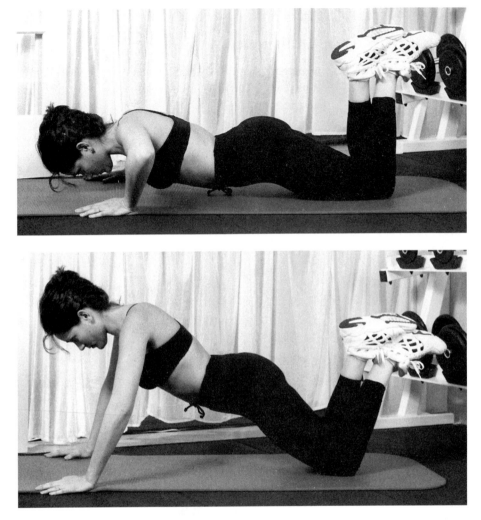

Lie on your stomach, legs together, hands pointing forward positioned under shoulders. Push up from the mat by fully straightening your elbows and using your knees as the pivotal point. You must keep your upper body in a straight line. Return to the starting position, chin to mat, without letting your stomach touch the mat. For support to keep from slipping, you may keep your lower legs flat against the mat, toes pointed.

Compare the number of push-ups that you completed successfully with the chart for the push-up test (p. 27).

Age (yrs)	15–19		20–29		30–39		40–49		50–59		60–69	
Gender	M	F	M	F	M	F	M	F	M	F	M	F
Excellent	>39	>33	>36	>30	>30	>27	>22	>24	>21	>21	>18	>17
Above Average	29–36	25–32	29–35	21–29	22–29	20–26	17–21	15–23	13–20	11–20	11–17	12–16
Average	23–28	18–24	22–28	15–20	17–21	13–19	13–16	11–14	10–12	7–10	8–10	5–11
Below Average	18–22	12–17	17–21	10–14	12–16	8–12	10–12	5–10	7–9	2–6	5–7	1–4
Poor	<17	<11	<16	<9	<11	<7	<9	<4	<6	<1	<4	<1

PERCENTILES

Age (yrs)	15–19		20–29		30–39		40–49		50–59		60–69	
Gender	M	F	M	F	M	F	M	F	M	F	M	F
Percentiles												
95	50	46	48	37	36	36	30	32	28	30	25	30
90	43	38	41	32	32	31	25	28	24	23	24	25
85	39	33	36	30	30	27	22	24	21	21	18	17
80	35	31	34	26	27	24	21	22	17	17	16	15
75	32	28	32	24	25	22	20	20	15	15	13	13
70	31	26	30	22	24	21	19	18	14	13	13	13
65	29	25	29	21	22	20	17	16	13	11	11	12
60	27	23	27	20	21	17	16	14	11	10	11	12
55	26	21	26	18	20	16	15	13	11	10	10	10
50	24	20	24	16	19	14	13	12	10	9	10	9
45	23	18	22	15	17	13	13	11	10	7	8	6
40	22	16	21	14	16	12	12	10	9	5	7	5
35	21	15	20	13	15	11	11	10	8	4	6	4
30	20	14	18	11	14	10	10	7	7	3	6	3
25	18	12	17	10	12	8	10	5	7	2	5	2
20	16	11	16	9	11	7	8	4	5	1	4	1
15	14	9	14	7	10	6	7	3	5	1	3	—
10	11	6	11	5	8	4	5	2	4	—	2	—
5	8	4	9	2	6	1	4	—	2	—	—	—

* Based on data from the Canada Fitness Survey, 1981

Reprinted by permission of the Canadian Society for Exercise Physiology.

Modified Sit and Reach

This test will measure your flexibility. You will need a yardstick and adhesive tape for this test. Place a yardstick on the floor with the zero mark closest to you. Tape the yardstick in place at the 15 inch mark. Ask a friend to help you to keep your legs straight during the test but be sure that your helper does not interfere with your movement.

Sit on the floor with the yardstick between your legs, feet 10 to 20 inches apart, and your heels even with the tape at the 15 inch mark. Place one hand over the other. The tips of your two middle fingers should be on top of one another. Slowly reach forward *without bouncing or jerking* and slide your fingertips along the yardstick as far as possible. The greater your reach, the higher your score will be.

Do the test three times, and record your best score to the nearest inch/inches.

Compare your score to the standards on this table:

MODIFIED SIT-AND-REACH

	Score at age				
	20–29	30–39	40–49	50–59	60+
MEN					
High	≥19	≥18	≥17	≥16	≥15
Average	13–18	12–17	11–16	10–15	9–14
Below average	10–12	9–11	8–10	7–9	6–8
Low	<9	<8	<7	<6	<5
WOMEN					
High	≥22	≥21	≥20	≥19	≥18
Average	16–21	15–20	14–19	13–18	12–17
Below average	13–15	12–14	11–13	10–12	9–11
Low	<12	<11	<10	<9	<8

Reprinted by permission from *ACSM Resource Manual for Guidelines for Exercise Testing and Prescription* (p. 165) by S. Blair, P. Painter, R.R. Pate, L.K. Smith, and C.B. Taylor, 1988, Philadelphia: Lea & Febiger, which was adapted from *The Y's Way to Physical Fitness* (pp. 106–111) by L.A. Golding, C.R. Myers, and W.E. Sinning (Eds.), 1982, Rosemont, IL: YMCA of the USA.

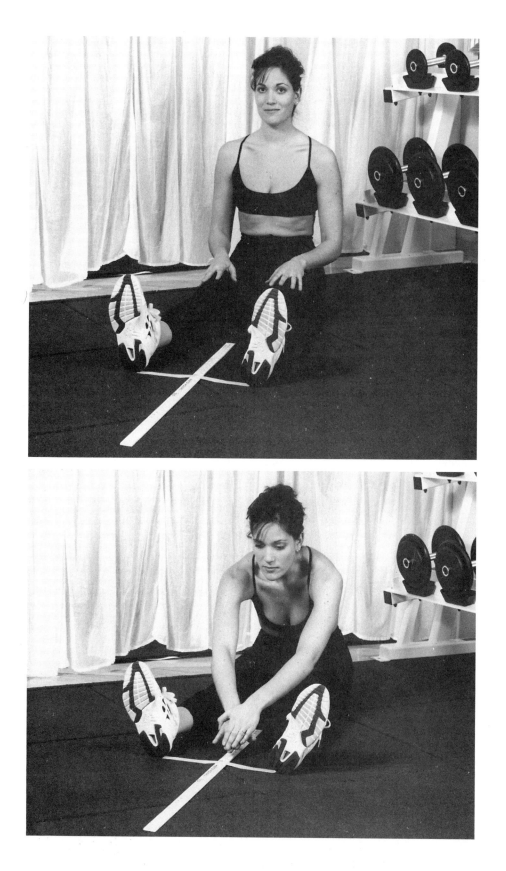

Exercise, moving, sweating, and breathing deeply are not unnatural acts. It's much more unnatural to sit in front of a TV for three or four hours straight. Still, we've adopted an attitude that says exercise might hurt you. Some people think you should see a doctor before you even take a walk.

Not true. It has been determined that if you use common sense and answer a few questions about your health beforehand, it's safe for you to begin a moderate to intense exercise program. The questionnaire below—Physical Activity Readiness or PAR-Q—should help you to determine if you're ready to start an exercise program. Remember to always listen to your body. And, if you experience any problems, don't hesitate to see your doctor.

PAR-Q & YOU

(A Questionnaire for People Aged 15 to 69)

Regular physical activity is fun and healthy, and increasingly more people are starting to become more active every day. Being more active is very safe for most people. However, some people should check with their doctor before they start becoming much more physically active.

If you are planning to become much more physically active than you are now, start by answering the seven questions below. If you are between the ages of 15 and 69, the PAR-Q will tell you if you should check with your doctor before you start. If you are over 69 years of age, and you are not used to being very active, check with your doctor.

Common sense is your best guide when you answer these questions. Please read the questions carefully and answer each one honestly: check YES or NO.

YES NO

☐ ☐ 1. Has your doctor ever said that you have a heart condition *and* that you should only do physical activity recommended by a doctor?

YES   NO

☐   ☐   2. Do you feel pain in your chest when you do physical activity?

☐   ☐   3. In the past month, have you had chest pain when you were not doing physical activity?

☐   ☐   4. Do you lose your balance because of dizziness or do you ever lose consciousness?

☐   ☐   5. Do you have a bone or joint problem that could be made worse by a change in your physical activity?

☐   ☐   6. Is your doctor currently prescribing drugs (for example, water pills) for your blood pressure or heart condition?

☐   ☐   7. Do you know of *any other reason* why you should not do physical activity?

If you answered:

YES *to one or more questions*

Talk with your doctor by phone or in person BEFORE you start becoming much more physically active or BEFORE you have a fitness appraisal. Tell your doctor about the PAR-Q and which questions you answered YES.

- You may be able to do any activity you want—as long as you start slowly and build up gradually. Or, you may need to restrict your activities to those which are safe for you. Talk with your doctor about the kinds of activities you wish to participate in and follow his/her advice.
- Find out which community programs are safe and helpful for you.

NO *to all questions*

If you answered NO honestly to *all* PAR-Q questions, you can be reasonably sure that you can:

- start becoming much more physically active—begin slowly and build up gradually. This is the safest and easiest way to go.
- take part in a fitness appraisal—this is an excellent way to determine your basic fitness so that you can plan the best way for you to live actively.

DELAY BECOMING MUCH MORE ACTIVE:

- If you are not feeling well because of a temporary illness such as a cold or a fever—wait until you feel better; or
- If you are or may be pregnant—talk to your doctor before you start becoming more active.

Please note: If your health changes so that you then answer YES to any of the above questions, tell your fitness or health professional. Ask whether you should change your physical activity plan.

© *Canadian Society for Exercise Physiology/Sociétè canadienne de physiologie de l'exercice.* Reprinted by permission.

A PEAK 10 BUDDY

I think Peak 10 partnerships are great, and I would recommend doing Peak 10 with a friend, or even someone who isn't yet a friend but who also wants to get into shape. You can motivate each other and help each other take measurements. An edge of competition can be very motivating too.

If you want to work out with someone, here are some tips. Find someone positive and committed. Ask yourself, honestly, if you can imagine this person successfully completing the program. Do you enjoy similar workouts? Can you agree on days and times to meet for regular measurement taking and pep talks? Above all, your buddy should be someone who can be supportive and get you back on track if you lose momentum.

Here is an example of two friends who did Peak 10 together. Marguerite is a medical editor in Manhattan and Ellen is a corporate communications writer from Brooklyn. Each took the other's before (and after) photographs. Although they worked out separately, they spoke every few days to check on their progress and feelings, and met every two weeks to take each other's measurements.

	Marguerite	Ellen
MEASUREMENTS:		
Neck	13¼"	12¾"
Shoulder	42"	37¾"
Chest	39¼"	36¼"
Waist	32¼"	27"
Hips	39½"	35"
Right thigh	24"	22"
Right calf	15½"	13¼"
Right upper arm	10¾"	11"
Right forearm	9½"	8½"
Height	5'6"	5'2"
Weight	150 lbs.	118 lbs.
Fat	30%	24%
TOTAL INCHES	226	203.25
Lean body mass	105 lbs.	90 lbs.
FITNESS TESTS:		
Push-ups	24 in 40 seconds	22 in 35 seconds
Modified sit and reach	16"	20"
Resting heart rate	80 beats/min.	64 beats/min.
Target Training Zone	140 to 179	133 to 177

The "total inches" line above is simply the sum of all the body measurements. As you lose body fat, this number will drop. It's just another way to chart your progress.

Also, at the very bottom you will see a "Target Training Zone" line. We will help you to determine your individual Target Training Zone in Chapter 5. As you can see, it differs according to training level and will change as you progress with the program.

CAROL'S STORY

Are you looking at your numbers and feeling a little discouraged? Here's some incentive. When my "star pupil" Carol first came to me, she wore—like almost everyone—black tights and a big T-shirt, doing a great job of fat camouflage. She didn't once look in the camera when I took her picture. Nor would she tell me how much she weighed. I didn't find out until she got on the scale. She's 5'6" and started Peak 10 at 176 pounds, 41.5 percent body fat, which translates to 61.88 pounds of fat and 103 pounds of lean muscle mass.

"I went to Chris because even though I had read all the magazine articles, bought all the books, and done all the diets, nothing ever worked," says Carol. "I realized that I needed special attention. I needed someone to focus on me."

Within ten days she was 166.5 pounds. Her body fat had changed about 2 percent. By the end of ten weeks, she was down to 141 pounds and 27.7 percent body fat. And she's still going strong.

ONE MORE THING

We've discussed—and will discuss further—what it's going to take to get your body into shape, but there's another part of your body that's along for the ride, and in reality it might be the most important part: Your mind. Your attitude. If your thinking is not positive, then Peak 10 might not work for you. No one else is going to care for your well-being the way you can. Everything you accomplish on Peak 10 is because you have a desire, the tools and the information you need, and because you honor your commitment. If any of these steps are a problem for you, I can offer some help.

I've explored a lot about what success means to me and my clients. While we all imagine the glory of having succeeded, we often try to ignore what scares us about success. Having unexamined feelings and thoughts about success can undermine our quest to complete a goal. So you and I have to consider what stops us from being as successful as we want to be.

Believe it or not, wanting to be thin isn't enough of a motivation for most people. I've found that people who are the most successful at Peak 10 don't do it simply to lose weight, but rather because they want to create a new focus and attitude about health. Instead, I hope my clients will work toward improving their relationship to food and exercise.

Likewise, if you simply exercise for the goal, and don't learn about your body and take part in all the steps of Peak 10, then you might not understand your body well enough to continue to improve it *after* Peak 10.

I hope to make exercise something you enjoy for itself or something that you do to get more enjoyment out of other activities. Taking care of your body—and of your mind—requires knowledge and energy, but if you see the process as work, rather than as a reward in and of itself, then I think Peak 10 will ultimately feel more difficult than it actually is.

It's not when a client tells me that she's lost five pounds that I feel good: It's when I hear, "I felt so good this weekend when I was with my family. I felt good in my clothes and I had enough energy to go biking with my kids, and after dinner, I didn't need to take two Alka-Seltzers." In other words, during and after Peak 10 you'll take good care of yourself because you will learn how. You deserve good health, confidence, and a high level of energy, so make sure that you do everything in your power to get it. All the tools are here.

And, to go one step further, a life of good health can translate into a good life in many ways. If you're not achieving greater excellence in all areas of your life, then chances are you're not living up to your potential. You're keeping yourself from your own success.

Look at your life. Are you someone who doesn't finish things, or doesn't allow yourself to feel all your feelings? Do you have trouble committing to your goals? Take a look at what this means. Does it show up in other areas of your life? What is the thread? What does it make you think of?

I don't want you to take part in Peak 10 because you believe you have to be miserable to have a nice body. That's not true, and that attitude doesn't allow for the fullness and enjoyment of life. You can begin to enjoy your body right now, no matter what you look like or what you think you should look like. You don't have to wait to feel good about yourself and to want the best out of life.

Peak 10 can serve as your first step toward fixing these difficulties in your life. My goal is to have Peak 10 strengthen your own sense of well-being. It goes beyond a total concept of what exercise should be, and brings balance into your life. If you can master this one step, this one program, then you can use this experience as a model to help you in other areas. This program will bring you excellence not because you'll look like Barbie or Ken, but because you'll be the best that you can be.

RICH'S STORY

I "woke up" one day and realized that I was a young man in an old man's body. Work had taken priority over my health and body, and if I kept up this pace things would only get worse. I found a way to make the time for exercise, because it was important to me, and it really started to pay off.

What I put *into* my body also became a priority. I really started to pay attention to what I ate, and cut out the red meat, cheese, and other really fattening things. I found that my diet could effect my body as much as weight training, if not more.

As my body began to change, so did my attitude. I felt better about myself, had more energy and wanted to work harder in the gym because of it. I'll never go back to the way I was. Now it's simple and easy to keep myself in good shape and I really enjoy it. All I have to do is take a look at my before pictures to remind myself what I have to loose . . . or should I say "gain."

Rich
Age: 28

Height: 5'9"	*Start*	*Finish*
MEASUREMENTS		
Neck	14.5	13.5
Shoulders	49	44.0
Chest	41.75	41.0
Waist	38.0	31.5
Hips	41.5	39.25
Rt. Thigh	24.75	23.0
Rt. Calf	15.75	14.5
Rt. Upper Arm	13.5	13.25
Rt. Forearm	11.5	10.5
Weight	193.5 lbs.	174.5 lbs.
% Fat	25.0	14.2
TOTAL INCHES	250.25	230.5

Inches lost: 19.75

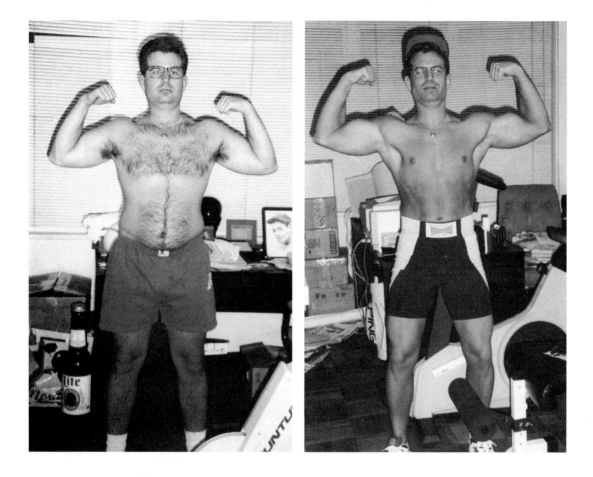

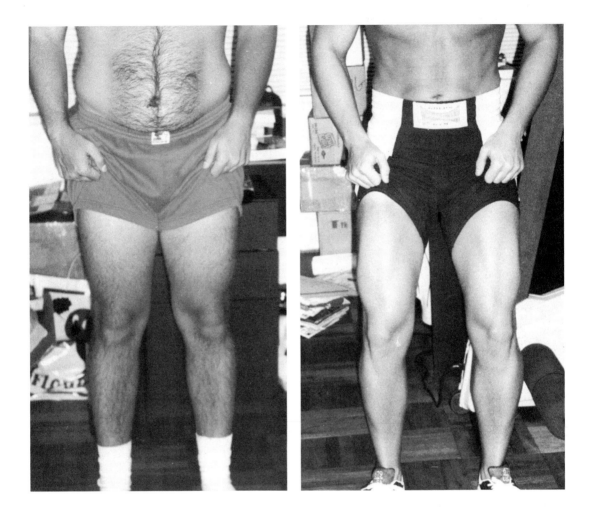

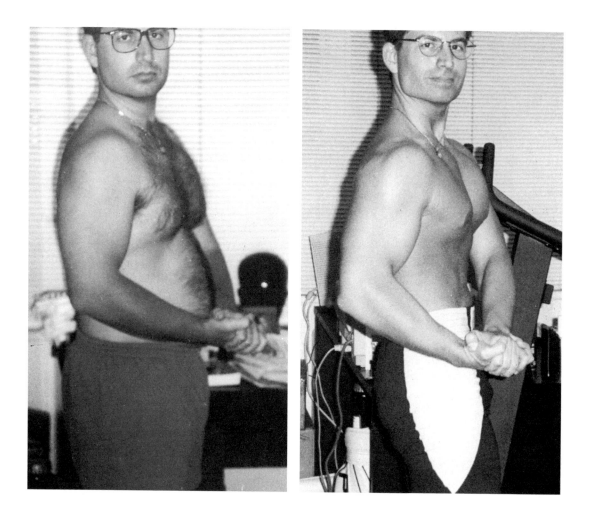

3

Eat to Peak

Over the years, we have all become familiar with use of the word *diet* to mean something we do to lose weight. A multibillion-dollar industry has been developed around it—we see it everywhere we look, and hear it in everyday conversation. Well, in this chapter and throughout this book, I'll refer to "diet" in its true sense. That is, according to Noah Webster: "what a person *usually* eats and drinks." It is this definition of "diet" that your nutritional plan must be built upon. You see, what we are going to do is change what you *usually* eat and drink, and in doing so we will change your body, your fitness level, and your life.

Eating foods that are high in fat and sugar on a consistent basis when you're involved in a regular exercise program will greatly reduce your progress. As a society, it is our regular diet of foods high in fat and processed sugars that contributes to the abundance of individuals fighting to be lean and more fit. On average we consume approximately 38 percent of our total calories in the form of fat and more than sixty pounds of table sugar annually. That's average. You might be better. You might be worse. The cumulative effect of this typical diet is over two million deaths each year from coronary heart disease alone. We're virtually killing ourselves.

I could go on and on about the miseries of being overfat and out of shape . . . from the physical consequences to the emotional challenges.

The result of an unhealthy lifestyle (fatty diet, low activity level, stress, drugs, alcohol, etc.) is a dramatically reduced potential.

There is no magic to the Peak 10 program. There is no special drink, no secret herb or pill. Like the other two components of the Peak 10 program, strength training and aerobic conditioning, the diet is based on:

1. Knowledge
2. Eating foods that promote a lean, strong, fit body
3. Moderation

You will learn that eating, along with its sensual and communal pleasures, is the process by which we fuel our bodies. I will take you through a day in the life of a Peakie (that's a person on Peak 10) to help you establish your own nutritional outline. Along the way I will provide you with enough information for you to take charge of what you *usually* eat and drink. Intelligently and with complete understanding, you will realize that the secrets and the magic of your success will come from you.

If you've taken the difficult road of "going on a diet," or even worse, you've binged and/or starved yourself, I'd like to reintroduce you to the world of food. Together we have to transform your dining habits slowly and gradually so that you can get used to a new, healthful way of eating. You don't need to "diet" to be thin; you need to *change* your diet and eat in a more healthful way.

Are you ready? Here we go!

ONE DAY ON THE PEAK 10 EATING PLAN (AND WHY IT WORKS)

Let me begin by telling you the basic guidelines for the Peak 10 eating plan. You will calculate your recommended daily caloric intake with my help. Then we will put together guidelines for you that allow for 15 percent of those calories to come from protein, 70 percent to come from carbohydrates, and 15 percent to come from fat.

The eating program is designed to be followed during the time that you are on Peak 10. The purpose of doing this is to establish your proper intake now, *and* for your new body. It is not designed to be followed forever, which would probably drive you and those around you nuts. Just know that by following it for ten weeks, you will help break yourself of some of the unhealthful habits that are now a part of your life.

Just as mother always said, you should be eating mostly vegetables and fruits. Everything else should be consumed less frequently and in smaller quantities. Grains, dairy products, and meats should likewise be consumed in smaller quantities. Even though bread is low in fat, you should pass up that bread basket while you're trying to lose fat—another one of those ancient tips that have turned out to be valid after all (more about that later). Now let's take a look at what your morning might be like.

THE MORNING

Because your new lifestyle commands so much energy, you wake up feeling hungry, and within an hour you've eaten a good nutritious, low-fat, high-fiber breakfast.

My Favorite Breakfast

1 serving of hot oatmeal (½ cup dry), with Equal, skim milk, and a dash of salt
1 apple
2 hard-boiled egg whites (Give the yolks to someone you don't like or just throw them out.)
1 large cup of mint tea
1 large glass of water with lemon

As far as I'm concerned (and other experts will agree), breakfast is the most important meal of the day. It has been anywhere from five to ten hours since you've eaten last and it's time to "break the fast."

Sitting down and taking the time to eat a complete healthful breakfast is a worthwhile investment for a high-energy, productive day. It jump-starts your metabolism and ignites the calorie-burning process. If you don't eat breakfast, your body will hold on to its energy supply—namely, fat. Eating breakfast stimulates calorie burning and can increase your metabolism. Don't worry if you don't like to eat immediately after getting up. Give yourself up to a couple of hours and then enjoy your breakfast—just be sure not to skip it! (See page 76 for more breakfast suggestions.)

CARBOHYDRATES

To rev up our engines each morning, you're going to eat a breakfast high in complex carbohydrates and full of vitamins, minerals, and fiber. For breakfast, these "carbs" generally come in the form of cereal and fresh fruit. Cereals and fruits, breads, grains, and vegetables are all sources of carbohydrates, but I usually prefer my vegetables later in the day.

Carbohydrates are the most abundant sources of energy. They are divided into two groups—the complex and the simple. Complex carbohydrates include starches and fibers. They are found in foods such as rice, grains, beans, and most vegetables. Because they are complex, they are broken down by our bodies and converted into the usable sugars that give us energy. The simple carbohydrates, or sugars, are found in many vegetables and fruits. Even milk products have their own simple sugar, called lactose. The most common and most abundant simple carbohydrate in our culture, however, is sucrose (table sugar). This stuff is in everything—especially now that most of the foods we eat are processed. Be on the lookout. (As a Peakie, your aim will be to consume fewer refined sugars.)

Your breakfast will also be high in fiber. Dietary fiber, a.k.a. bulk or roughage, will become your new best friend, your bodyguard of sorts. Fiber is an essential element in our diet, even though it provides no nutrients at all. Fiber is the indigestible materials found in plants. Chewing it stimulates saliva flow, and the bulk it adds in the stomach and intestines during digestion provides more time for the absorption of nutrients. Sorry to bring this up at breakfast, but diets with sufficient fiber permit bowel regularity (this is a very healthful thing) and help you avoid constipation and other more serious intestinal disorders. Fiber also helps fill you up, so you feel satisfied. Eating fruits, vegetables, legumes, whole-grain breads, and low-fat products made from bran and oats will give you the dietary fiber you desperately need.

Chris—

It's all your fault.

I'm mellllting.
Wow, a whole new me . . . and the fans are starting to notice.

Wasa bread is my new fiber friend. We're gettin' along just fine. Yes, I'm more regular . . .

The other night I got home (to my new home) and I was hungry and feelin' good, and there they were, those chips some of my "helpers" brought in on moving night, so I grabbed them . . . Then this bell went off and, wham, I thought these just aren't worth it! So I put the chips back and went to my full fruit bowl and crunched on an apple while I got dinner started.

Anyway, I really think I'm on the road to a whole new life with food. I admit I still use olive oil sometimes and I'm far from perfect but this is really working!

A million thanks for including me and getting me pointed in a direction that has a future!

Anne

PROTEIN

To get some of the protein you need every day try a veggie-filled egg-white omelette (hey, there's a way to fit vegetables into breakfast!), cooked up in a nonstick pan (Egg Beaters omelettes are great too), or try skim milk that you add to your cereal. Protein is critically important and will make up approximately 15 percent of the total calories you consume in the day.

The word "protein" originally meant "of prime importance." This doesn't mean that you should eat only protein, but that proteins are the building blocks of *all* life. Protein-rich foods from animal sources include fish, chicken and turkey, beef, and pork as well as milk and eggs. They contain complete proteins, or the essential amino acids our bodies need and cannot make themselves. No plants or grains contain whole proteins, so vegetarians must combine foods (such as beans and rice) to get the proper complement of amino acids.

Proteins play a role in virtually every cellular function. For instance, they regulate muscle contraction, antibody production, healing, muscle maintenance, and blood vessel expansion and contraction to maintain normal blood pressure. Generally, a lack of protein in the diet can retard normal growth in children and can cause a decrease in your overall energy level.

"Keep It Clear"

It's very important to give fluids to your body when you first wake up. You weigh less in the morning and have darker-colored urine because your body has lost water throughout the night.

It might be difficult to get into the habit, but plain old water is just what your body wants and needs first thing in the morning. Herbal teas, hot or cold, are also good choices. If you can't break your morning habit of a caffeine-filled cup of coffee or tea to get you started, that's fine, as long as you water up shortly after, since the caffeine is a diuretic and will cause your body to lose water.

Even if you don't feel "thirsty," you still need fluids. Don't rely on your senses to tell you when you are dehydrated, for they can be wrong. Use the color of your urine as a true indicator for your water needs. As I tell my clients, "Keep it clear." Eight to ten 8-ounce glasses each day should do it, but feel free to drink more. It's nearly impossible to overdo it.

Fat Rap

Of course, early in the morning it's hard to remember why you need protein, carbohydrates, and fiber. You'll just want to eat something that tastes good and is relatively easy to make. At times it's more convenient to grab coffee and a donut, but eating like this cheats your body in a couple of ways. Along with the obvious lack of nutritional value, this kind of "quickie" breakfast derives most of its calories from fat.

Now, let's talk fat, a "fat rap" of sorts. A calorie describes a measurement of heat or energy. Every food has a caloric value, which is equal to the amount of energy it provides, just like logs for a fire. Protein and carbohydrates provide 4 calories per gram, while fat provides 9 calories.

When you eat 10 grams of protein (about three egg whites) or 10 grams of carbohydrates (about one-third of a cup of cooked oatmeal), you consume 40 calories. On the other hand, if you eat 10 grams of fat (less than one tablespoon of butter), you kick back 90 calories. It's easy to see that fat is pretty concentrated stuff. And just like anything concentrated, you have to use it sparingly.

Fat is the Dr. Jekyll and Mr. Hyde of nutrients. Despite its evil reputation, fat does serve a valuable purpose in our bodies. It is one of those things we can't live without, but take it for granted and it can come around and bite you in the butt. Fat does provide us with a steady source of slow-burning energy, about 9 calories per gram. While reading this book you are burning around 50 percent of your total calories in the form of fat. Unfortunately, just reading this book won't make you lean. Fat just happens to be the fuel of choice when the body is at rest. Increasing your lean muscle mass and being more fit will help you burn even more fat calories at rest, as much as 80 to 90 percent more (which will happen if you stick to the program).

Another function of fat is that it helps to regulate some of the body's chemical needs: One in particular is maintaining our sex hormones. You just knew sex and fat had to be related somewhere along the line, didn't you? Fat also carries certain essential vitamins such as A, D, E, and K. Don't panic: It only takes about 20 grams each day to move these vitamins, the equivalent of about one and a half tablespoons of olive oil. For smaller people, 20 grams might be more fat than what you will be shooting for as your *total* daily fat consumption. And don't forget that when it comes to energy, your body could also use some of that stuff that you already have stored—which is the whole idea, right?

Anything else? Fat insulates our nerves, allowing them to function. It also surrounds our vital organs and joints to help protect them from injury. Since most fat is stored just beneath the skin, it helps to regulate our body temperature. People with a lot of body fat can generally withstand cooler temperatures, while very lean people are more susceptible to the cold.

Fat has its purpose, and because we can't live without it, nature has made sure we always want it. Why do you think it tastes so *good*? Understanding why we need fat and that most of us already have plenty stored can help you better regulate your intake. We also need to understand that we are all challenged by the adaptations that have helped us survive thousands of years as a species, through times when food wasn't nearly as plentiful as it is today. Given a leaner, more nutritious diet and of course time, our bodies will establish a better set point for both lean mass and fat storage. In other words, your body can re-adapt and begin to store less fat.

So you've had a satisfying breakfast. You feel full, but you don't feel tired. And the greatest part is that your breakfast was low in fat, so you boosted your metabolism without contributing to the fat that you already have stored.

YOUR METABOLISMS

Boost your metabolism? We've all heard of this thing called a metabolism. Some individuals feel that theirs doesn't exist. The truth is, not only does every living person have a metabolism, but we happen to have *three*.

In general, a metabolism is the sum of all the chemical reactions that take place in our bodies that are used for the production of work. Metabolism here means the rate at which our bodies produce energy.

The most common, or basic, is called the *basal metabolism*. This is the minimal amount of energy required to keep us alive—that is, the energy required to support muscle contraction for breathing, heartbeat, and muscle tone, as well as the maintenance of the continuous processes that occur in our cells. In general, a woman's basal metabolism burns about 1,200 calories a day, while a man's burns about 1,500 a day.

Fortunately, you can increase these numbers. The most effective way to raise your basal metabolism is to increase your lean body mass—the amount of muscle you have—because muscles burn calories faster than fat does. So if your body is more muscular, you will burn more calories throughout the day. Translation? A 180-pound person with 20 percent body fat burns more calories than a 180-pound person who has 35 percent body fat. So once again, muscles use more calories than fat does.

Active metabolism measures the energy you use for activities above and beyond living, such as walking, talking, laughing, carrying something, cooking dinner, working at a computer, running, or taking a shower. It's the energy you burn above and beyond what your body uses to function. Just as our food has caloric values, so do the activities we take part in. Running for one hour can expend from 620 to 900 calories, while doing light housework might use 250 calories in an hour. The more active you are, the more calories you will burn above and beyond the basic 1,200 or 1,500 calories each day.

Oh! That reminds me. Eating is on the active metabolism list because eating and digestion require energy. How ironic is that? We burn additional calories when we eat and then afterward as well. The point is, when you eat infrequently or not at all, you cause your metabolism to slow down. Any kind of prolonged period you go without eating, your body's internal engine slows down. By skipping breakfast, or in fact, skipping any meal, you will hinder your metabolism. This pattern of eating is not the way to become lean.

The third type of metabolism is referred to as the *thermoregulatory system*. Briefly, this system maintains and adjusts your body's temperature according to the surroundings. It also helps us to expend excess calories as heat. It is another way that the body works to maintain balance. A more physically fit person will have a thermoregulatory system that will burn more additional calories that we don't need than the system of someone who is unfit. Yet another advantage to being fit.

SNACKTIME

Okay, let's continue through our Peak 10 day. It's been about three hours since you've eaten breakfast. Maybe you've been at work or running errands and you didn't even notice that you're hungry. Your Dietary Recall says you should have a midmorning snack, such as fig bars, yogurt, or an apple, but why do you need to eat so soon after breakfast? Well, in order to keep your metabolism high, you must eat consistently throughout the day. I'll explain.

Your body creates some of the energy it needs by turning carbohydrates, fats, and protein into forms of sugar which are burned as fuel. The rate at which we use these foods as fuel is our metabolism. If you don't put fuel (food) into your body, then your metabolism slows down. In fact, to compensate for the lack of fuel it is receiving, your body begins to hold on to its fat— just in case it needs some energy later. So if you don't eat throughout the day, your body stops burning any unnecessary calories as soon as possible.

Now, let's say you're *starving* when snacktime rolls around. That's okay too. Becoming more active signals your body to burn more calories, which causes your appetite to increase. All this is normal and healthy, but you've got to keep it in check like everything else. That is why it is so important to take the time and make the effort for a snack, because if you don't, you will be even more hungry later, and more susceptible to overeating or making a bad food choice. Just keep eating high-fiber, low-fat foods (less than 15 percent of total calories from fat) and you'll become an incredible fat-burning machine. Fruit of any kind is the perfect snack—easy to carry, easy to keep in your purse, backpack, or briefcase. Nonfat yogurt is also a great nutritious treat that you can take on the go. Enjoy it!

SUPER SNICKYSNACKS

(a little heartier for when you're *really* hungry)

- Chopped apple with nonfat vanilla sugar-free yogurt on top
- Carrots and celery with Chris's Easy Dip
- Two handfuls of pretzels with Chris's Easy Dip
- ¼ cantaloupe with nonfat cottage cheese

Chris's Easy Dip

1 8-oz. container nonfat plain yogurt
½ packet powdered beef or vegetable bouillon or low-sodium bouillon
1 tsp. Worcestershire sauce
1 tsp. finely chopped onion
pepper to taste
Combine all ingredients and mix thoroughly.

If you're *not* craving a snack at this point in the day, reevaluate your last twelve to twenty-four hours. Did you have breakfast? Was it low in fat? Did you get enough sleep? Are you "keeping it clear"? What did you have for dinner last night? Before your body turns on its autopilot, and living a balanced life becomes second nature, you need to be asking yourself questions and practicing the lifestyle of someone who's lean and fit. In just a couple of days you will understand which patterns keep you from achieving your health goals. We are all different and we all have different needs, but as I said earlier, in order to be your physical best, the daily blueprint you follow will always translate directly into the way you look and feel.

What does that mean? It means that if you're skipping lunch or not drinking enough water or even if you're not taking the time to exercise sometime during the day, then you probably aren't feeling as well as you'd like to. Change your habits and you will change your life.

What are some habits to change? Hopefully, you're taking the stairs instead of the elevator. You're walking to the market instead of driving. In terms of food, the piece of fruit or cup of yogurt you had as a midmorning snack saved you from a midday craving for a high-fat, high-sugar lunch. Try reaching for the crudite rather than the potato chips at a party. Enjoy the sensation of going to sleep a little bit hungry rather than stuffed to the gills. Every candy bar that you pass up is a personal victory that will move you closer to your goal. All you need to do is to become more aware of what you are eating . . . And one way to do that is to always read labels. In fact, why don't we learn how to read a food label right now?

HOW TO READ A FOOD LABEL

You probably stand in front of the peanut butter jars in the supermarket thinking, "Which one should I pick?" (Actually, I hope you're staying away from peanut butter altogether, but this is just an example.) Since one jar says, "New! Lower in fat!" you turn it around to see how much more healthful it is. Isn't peanut butter fattening? You try to figure out the label: "Percent Daily Value" and fat grams. What do they mean?

SAMPLE NUTRITION FACTS

Reduced-Fat Peanut Butter

Serving Size 2 Tbs.
Servings Per Container about 14
Calories 190 / Fat Calories 108

AMOUNT/ SERVING	%DV	AMOUNT/ SERVING	%DV
Total Fat 12g	18%	Total Carb. 15g	5%
Sat Fat 2.5g	12%	Dietary Fiber 2g	8%
Cholest. 0mg	0%	Sugars 4g	
Sodium 250mg	10%	Protein 8g	

Regular Peanut Butter

Serving Size 2 Tbs.
Servings Per Container about 11
Calories 190 / Fat Calories 144

AMOUNT/ SERVING	%DV	AMOUNT/ SERVING	%DV
Total Fat 16g	25%	Total Carb. 7g	2%
Sat Fat 3g	16%	Dietary Fiber 2g	9%
Cholest. 0mg	0%	Sugars 4g	
Sodium 150mg	6%	Protein 8g	

To help consumers understand exactly what they are getting when they choose certain foods, the Food and Drug Administration recently changed the information labels that must appear on all food packaging. Unfortunately, it isn't that easy to figure out the labels that are supposed to be extra helpful. And in some cases, we are more confused than before they "fixed" the labels.

You picked up that jar of peanut butter because it said "lower in fat," but compared to what? Today, foods that say "low fat" or "reduced calories" or even "healthy" (even if it's in the *title* of the food, such as Healthy Choice frozen foods) must meet certain standards set by the FDA. You can be sure that such foods do not exceed certain levels for total fat, saturated fat, cholesterol, and sodium. The food must also meet minimum levels for some other nutrients. But there are still ways for the manufacturer to sidestep these standards by saying something is "lower in fat" than it was before, because that doesn't necessarily mean that it is *low* in fat. And remember, the standards are set by the FDA, so in some ways they are more relaxed than the standards that you will uphold throughout Peak 10.

A serving size, which is usually on the left side of the information label, now more accurately reflects a true serving. It used to be that a potato chip manufacturer could declare three potato chips to be a serving. But who eats only three potato chips? Today, the FDA determines exactly what a serving is. So check the package. How many cookies are in a serving? How much pasta is in a serving? How much cereal? Check the label and see how much you're eating. Even now that the portions have been recalculated, you might still be accustomed to eating more than the typical portion size.

To be sure that you know what your portions should look like, measure them out for three days and put them in your dishes to see what a portion looks like. Do this for everything that you eat until you are familiar with portion sizes.

Learn to count fat grams. The good news? Even if the small servings are hard to believe, at least you can figure out how much fat you're eating, and that's a great way to eat better balanced meals. The new labels must list the number of fat grams in one serving. If you know how many fat grams you should eat each day (which we will calculate later in the chapter), then it's very easy to use the labels to help you count.

"Percent Daily Value" is where it gets confusing. The regular peanut butter has 16 grams of fat per serving, and the label says that those grams equal 25 percent of your daily value. That might not sound so bad to you.

The FDA has assumed it knows how many calories make up your eating plan—2,000 a day with 30 percent coming from fat. With Peak 10, we will establish your *personal* daily caloric requirements, and only *15* percent of those calories should be coming from fat. So you see, that serving of peanut butter might be all the fat that you should have in one day. And do you know what that means? If you eat it, you're going to go over your limit by the end of the day.

You see, most everything that we put into our mouths has at least scant amounts of fat. Combine these tiny quantities over the course of a day, adding in the fat in your water-packed tuna or your grilled chicken breast, and you'll see that without any added fat in cooking or preparation, you still get enough fat in a day to keep your body functioning well and to get on the right track to becoming lean.

Remember, too, that the Percent Daily Value is based on the FDA's idea of a serving. If you're eating more than the two tablespoons of peanut butter, then you're eating a larger percentage of your daily value.

Sample Nutrition Facts

Light Mayonnaise

Serving Size 1 Tbs.
Servings Per Container about 32
Calories 50 / Fat Calories 45

Amount/ Serving	%DV	Amount/ Serving	%DV
Total Fat 5g	8%	Total Carb. 1g	0%
Sat Fat 1g	4%	Protein 0g	
Cholest. 5mg	2%	Sodium 115mg	10%

Nonfat Mayonnaise

Serving Size 1 Tbs.
Servings Per Container about 32
Calories 10 / Fat Calories 0

Amount/ Serving	%DV	Amount/ Serving	%DV
Total Fat 0g	0%	Total Carb. 2g	1%
Sat Fat 0g	0%	Protein 0g	
Cholest. 0mg	0%	Sodium 105mg	6%

Above are two labels, one for fat-free mayonnaise and one for low-fat mayo. Take a look at the difference, and you will see that there can be a great advantage to picking fat-free foods if you take the time to read the labels and really understand what you're eating. This nonfat mayo is a great choice to lubricate your tuna salad.

To determine fat intake, I prefer to count actual grams rather than using the Percent Daily Value (%DV) column. But to simplify things, you can limit your fat intake by never eating anything with more than 15 or 20 percent fat. The complicated thing is that this is *not* the same number as the %DV that is on labels. Most labels tell you the fat calories per serving, but not the percentage of fat from calories per serving. Here is the calculation from the top: Fat grams times 9 equals fat calories. Total calories divided by fat calories equals the percentage of fat.

Let's take peanut butter, since we're already in that aisle. In the regular peanut butter there are 16 fat grams per serving. I multiply that by 9 and get 144 (fat calories per serving). Then I take the fat calories per serving (144) and divide it by the total calories (190), which makes the total fat of this peanut butter 76 percent. Whether you eat the recommended serving or dip your finger and lick it, this *percentage* of fat from calories stays the same. Now, if you are keeping your fat under 15 percent, this doesn't even come close. And, just so you have a basis of comparison, let's calculate the percentage of fat in the reduced-fat peanut butter: 12 grams of fat multiplied by 9 is 108 fat calories. Divide that by 190, which is the total calories, and you get 57 percent. Still way too high for someone who wants to be lean.

Sugar, Fat's Evil Twin

Let's not forget fat's evil twin, sugar. The two often come together and create a nightmare for people trying to stay fit. When I think of the combination of fat and sugar, I remember Violet. She was the little (or should I say portly) girl from *Willie Wonka and the Chocolate Factory* who ate something that she wasn't supposed to and blew up to enormous proportions. Well, in a way that's what the combination of fat and sugar will do to you. Sugar has the ability to stimulate fat cells, enabling them to suck up the free-floating fat. If you boost your blood lipid level by eating something that the typical overfat person normally eats, like a milkshake (with a burger) or ice cream (with that cake), guess where the sugar goes? You got it! Right into the fat cell, making it nice and plump, giving you those bumpy contours we all hate. Yep, it's that extra fat in the fat cell that pushes it over the limit. So even though that chocolate syrup is fat-free and always has been, that doesn't mean that it won't make you fat. "Fat-free" is not the promise of good health that we've been led to believe.

You have to watch the entire content of what you eat, not just the fat, because even the misuse of sugar can increase the amount of fat on your body. Look for foods that are low in both fat *and* sugar. Avoid those "fat-free" cookies and desserts. While they may be low in fat, they are packed full of sugar. If you read a few labels, you'll see that there are about 50 calories (five minutes of jogging) in just one of those measly fat-free cookies. And if you're like most people, you have to eat even *more* fat-free cookies to satisfy your craving.

Food labels must now include a list of all the sugars found in the food. (On labels, sugar also appears as sucrose or corn syrup.) But you need to know that not all sugars are alike. For example, a label for milk lists sugar and so does a label for M&M's. The FDA does not require manufacturers to say whether the sugar occurs naturally (such as in milk) or is added in processing (as in the M&M's). But sugar isn't sugar isn't sugar. The sugar in milk is complemented by calcium, protein, and other vitamins and minerals. The sugar in the M&M's is accompanied by chocolate! Yummy, but not nearly as healthful as skim milk.

The most healthful foods have no labels. Apples, broccoli, potatoes, spinach. No one is labeling these healthful, but you know that they're good for you. In general, fresh fruits and vegetables are the best sources of vitamins and minerals—and they are mostly fat-free.

Fresh is always better. Fresh chicken, fish, and beef are more nutritional and less fatty than their processed counterparts. And be aware that labels that say "low in fat" or "reduced sodium" are comparing themselves to other foods in that category, not to other food in general. For instance, one brand of smoked turkey dogs may be lower in fat than another, but that doesn't mean that the turkey dogs are more healthful than a couple slices of fresh turkey. They most definitely are not.

LUNCHTIME

You've eaten breakfast and a small snack and you feel great, strong, and have lots of energy. You might be planning to "do lunch" with a friend or perhaps take a break from a project and grab a quick bite to eat. You opt for a meal that's simple and light. A meal that won't slow you down twenty minutes after it left your plate. You want to eat a healthful lunch. What might that be?

THE *REAL* POWER LUNCH

Skip the martinis! If you're out for a power lunch, self-discipline is the way to impress them. Broiled fish or chicken, sans sauce. Some fresh or steamed veggies with balsamic vinegar or mustard sauce. A plain baked potato. Fresh berries in season and herbal tea or decaffeinated coffee to top it all off. There's nothing like control and working yourself into your best shape possible to get confidence.

Knock 'em dead!

As with all your meals, lunch will be high in complex carbohydrates, with a moderate amount of protein and a small amount of fat. It helps to think of lunch as a meal, rather than something to fill you up until dinner. I realize that you are probably eating between meetings or in the middle of a busy day, but it's very important to take the time to eat a healthful, filling meal. Some of the best lunch choices include hearty vegetable or bean soup combined with a lean sandwich of turkey or tuna (in water, not oil) stuffed with all the veggies you can fit between two slices of whole-wheat or other whole-grain bread; mixed greens and veggies with a small amount of grilled chicken or fish topped with low-fat or nonfat dressing; beans with rice topped with a wonderful tomato salsa. All these choices make lunch a power refill and not the fat-storing dilemma that most people experience. Take a "pass" when your office-mates order fried chicken with mashed potatoes and artery-clogging gravy. Most sandwich places will make a chicken or turkey sandwich with no mayo and lots of veggies. Or if that doesn't work for you, take time the night before to pack a lunch. Make your own healthful sandwich just the way you like it.

AFTERNOON SNACKTIME

The day is really flying by. Before you turned your life around with Peak 10, you probably hit the wall at around four o'clock and wondered if anyone had bottled energy for sale.

If your gas tank is on "E," you might have an urge for some fatty, sugary, ultrasatisfying snack—maybe a candy bar with enough fat and sugar to send you to the moon. Eat it and you will have eaten a food that has no nutritional value, which won't help you when you want to exercise tomorrow.

So, for your late afternoon snack, I suggest a piece of fruit, a glass of juice with a few pretzels, some yogurt, tomato juice or V-8, or some raw veggies. Remember, don't skip your snack. Eating less frequently will not help you lose weight or body fat. It will only cause your metabolism to slow down, and come dinner, you'll be so hungry you could lose control. A light healthful snack and a little movement are just what you need to give you a little afternoon boost. And if that doesn't work, maybe tea or coffee is in order.

We sometimes mistake boredom or tiredness for hunger. We eat to pick ourselves up, even though it's not really food that we crave. If you do feel tired or bored, find another solution besides food. Stand outside for a few minutes while you eat your apple. Work on something that doesn't require a lot of concentration. If you find yourself continuously eating poorly at this time of day, have a healthful snack and try to think of a creative solution to avoid the urge to eat something fattening and unhealthful. Pay attention to your energy level and, if possible, arrange your day accordingly.

Avoid the 4 p.m. Snack Pit

- Make unhealthful food inaccessible during that time.
- Schedule an appointment to keep you occupied.
- Plan errands after lunch during the afternoon doldrums.
- Plan to exercise then.
- Keep only healthful snacks around.

Cocktail Hour

It's nearing cocktail hour, and maybe you really enjoy a drink or two in the evening. Without passing judgment on any of the social ramifications of a drink, I would like to simply explain how alcohol affects a Peakie. If you are truly serious about getting into great shape, and I will assume that you are, then the most important thing for you to know about alcohol is that I don't recommend that you drink it while you are on Peak 10. Alcohol has no fat, but lots of empty calories. So if you drink you are using up valuable calories with something that has no vitamins or minerals or protein—nothing to help your body rebuild itself, nothing to keep it functioning. Those calories are prime candidates to be recruited for your ever-thirsty fat cells. And at 100 to 200 or more calories a pop, drinks can really add up.

Another adverse effect of alcohol consumption is that it impairs your judgment—just ask those test dummies. Even if you escape an accident with a car, you might have an accident with a loaded refrigerator—not as destructive initially, but over time it can be deadly.

WHAT'S IN A DRINK?

Here are some calorie counts for popular drinks:

12 oz. beer	146 calories
12 oz. light beer	100 calories
piña colada	262 calories
screwdriver	174 calories
whiskey sour	138 calories
wine spritzer	85 calories
3½ oz red wine	74 calories
3½ oz white wine	70 calories
rum cocktail	109 calories
3½ oz. champagne	62 calories
Bloody Mary	116 calories
Daquiri	111 calories
frozen Daquiri	185 calories
Gin & tonic	171 calories
Manhattan	128 calories
Margarita	189 calories
Martini	156 calories

I do occasionally enjoy a glass of red wine or beer. But the key is *occasionally*, and I want you to know that the more alcohol you consume, the slower your progress in this program will be. Alcohol is the first thing that I cut out when I want to get in especially good shape for a particular event. So please, use your good judgment and really evaluate what is most important to you.

DINNERTIME

Finally! Dinnertime. You have maintained your energy throughout the day. In fact, you're probably not as hungry as you used to be. That's a great feeling, especially when that bread basket comes out at the restaurant. Or when you're preparing a meal at home and you usually snack your way through three courses before dinner is even served.

Congratulations are in order. Do you see what you've done? You've made the right choices and eaten more healthful food throughout the day—and come dinnertime, you possess the control to resist your former unhealthful pattern of eating. You are less prone to eat what most unfit and overfat people would eat. *You ate. You have control. That's what it's all about.*

When it comes time to make choices for dinner, it should be light and nutritious, preferably earlier in the evening, so that you have plenty of time to digest and use those calories.

Comfort-Food Dinner

1 serving of low-fat vegetable, chicken noodle, or minestrone soup
Calories 80; protein 7g; carbs 10g; fat 2g
1 low-fat grilled cheese sandwich:
2 slices of whole-grain bread (90–100 calories, 2g fat per slice)
2 slices of fat-free Swiss cheese (30 calories, 0g fat per slice)
3 slices of fresh tomato (about 5 calories per slice)
Cooking spray on outside of bread (9 calories, 1g fat)
Calories 289; protein 18g; carbs 47g; fat 5g

Let's examine the typical 1990s American dinner. Soup, salad, bread, appetizer, entree, dessert—the choices are endless. And our habits as a society are rooted in overindulgence. It has become part of family life for many.

Sometimes I imagine the "traditional" family coming home after a hard day of work and school. Mom and Dad and their three kids don't want to wait around for dinner—and no one wants to cook dinner—so they all head off to McDonald's or another fast-food restaurant. And who can blame them? After a long hard day, buying groceries and creating a healthful meal require a lot of energy, energy that most of us would rather spend enjoying our family and friends, right? But at what cost do you drop into a fast-food restaurant?

A double cheeseburger is 680 calories. French fries are 230. A hot apple pie comes in at 280, which totals the meal up to 1,190 calories—and that's with a *diet* soda! That's way too many calories for one meal, not to mention all that fat. Your body doesn't stand a chance if you eat this stuff regularly.

Tips for Dining Out

- Decide what you will eat before you get to the restaurant.
- Ask for a fresh vegetable platter instead of the customary bread "pacifier."
- Take charge. Ask the kitchen to prepare items to your specifications. For example, order a piece of fish broiled without butter, with extra lemon on the side. Most restaurants are used to this and will be cooperative. (If they're not, you might try restaurants that are more cooperative.)
- Ask to have items prepared with lemon, lime, wine, mustard, or meatless tomato sauce.
- Avoid ordering red meat, but if you must, make sure you limit your portions.
- Trim excess fat or skin from meat, fish, and poultry.

Healthful fast food? It's not easy to find. But here are a few examples of what we eat when we're too pooped to do our own cooking:

1. Chinese food: We order steamed vegetables with white-meat chicken, no sauce, and brown rice. For a treat we get steamed vegetable dumplings and a small helping of hot-and-sour soup. (Skip this if you're trying to avoid sodium.)
2. Pizza: We order our pizza prepared with little or no cheese, fresh tomato, and mushrooms or spinach. If we order cheeseless, we add some grated fat-free mozzarella and a sprinkle of Parmesan and stick it back in the oven for five minutes.
3. Sushi: California rolls are great, without the risks of raw fish if that bothers you. Also, they make great salads at Japanese restaurants (skim the oil off the ginger dressing, and only use a small amount of it, or use your own fat-free dressing). Miso soup is low-fat and delicious too.

Carol's Story (continued)

I worked out a Peak 10 plan that was aggressive and realistic. Chris pushed me, but not beyond myself. Even though I had 30-plus pounds to lose, I didn't burn out. I ate inconsistently before I met Chris and I was attempting to burn fat above my anaerobic threshold, which I now know is inefficient.

Carol Age: 29 Height: 5'6"	*Start*	*Finish*
MEASUREMENTS		
Neck	13.25	12.50
Shoulders	41.50	39.25
Chest	39.0	34.50
Waist	33.75	28.50
Hips	43.75	38.50
Rt. Thigh	27.0	23.5
Rt. Calf	15.75	14.75
Rt. Upper Arm	14.0	12.00
Rt. Forearm	9.50	8.75
Weight	176.5 lbs.	142.5 lbs.
% Fat	41.0	26.25
TOTAL INCHES	237.50	212.25

Inches lost: 25.25

The heart monitor helped me immediately. It helped me see that I had not been burning as much fat as I could have. Also, I had never lifted weights before. Chris always gets me to do three or five more reps. You know what he always says? "Just keep going to failure, babe. . . ." My weight training workouts with Chris were intense. Even though the training hour was grueling, afterward I felt exhilarated.

I started my first Peak 10 when I was 29. I did Peak 10 in the fall and then stopped for the holidays. I maintained everything and didn't go on any binges. Peak 10 enhanced my life.

I wrote down the things that would help me stick to the program, because each person needs something different and something special. I'm a private person and I don't like to talk too much. Peak 10 was a personal thing for me. I told my family, who were supportive and wonderful, but I didn't tell my friends. I would eat before I went out with them and just say I wasn't hungry or I would simply ask for exactly what I wanted, such as grilled chicken over a green salad without dressing.

Chris is so cute. He always said "Keep it clear" to make sure I was drinking enough water and "Ya bundle up" if I complained about it being too cold to go for a walk. Chris has lots of ways of saying "Just do it," but

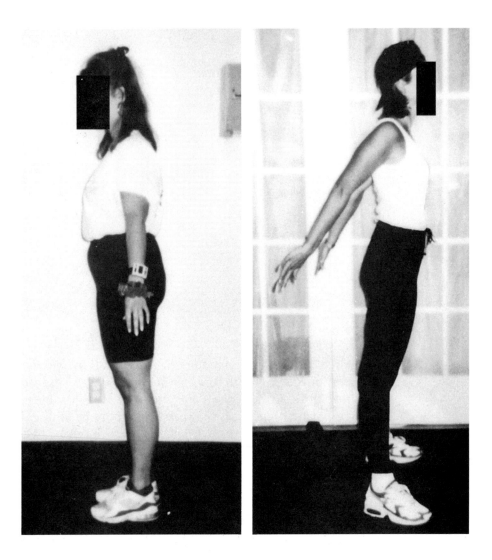

the truth is, you have to find what works for you, just like I had to find what works for me.

After I finished my first Peak 10, it was so successful that I decided to do it again because I was already on a roll. Once I got accustomed to the way I should be eating, I had more energy left over to focus on turning up the intensity of my workouts. The photos on the right are after two Peak 10s, the measurements are after one. As you can see I'm a different person. And I feel great!

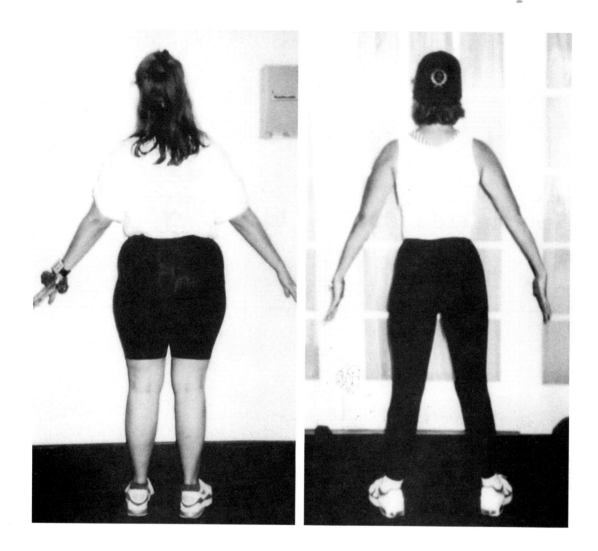

4

Creating Your Balanced Diet

On the Peak 10 eating plan you will eat a balanced diet in which approximately 15 percent of your total calories for the day are in the form of lean protein, 70 percent carbohydrates, and 15 percent fat (mostly unsaturated). That translates to approximately:

70% carbohydrates = vegetables, fruits, and grains
15% protein = fish, poultry, meat, milk/dairy, legumes
15% fat = occurs naturally in most proteins and some carbohydrates

Don't worry if on some days you have three grains and only one milk. The point, as always, is balance. To simplify things, I'm going to give you some lists to choose from to get the proper balance of foods.

Remember, one of the most important parts of your eating plan is water. You need to drink a minimum of eight 8-ounce glasses of water every day plus 8 oz for every 20 minutes of exercise to replace the fluid you'll lose. And even if you're not exercising, it's still important to drink water.

All the foods you eat—whether in your house or at a restaurant—should be prepared without added fat. Most foods have enough fat to provide flavor, and there are various ways to cook food without using oil or butter. Try steaming, grilling, and broiling your food. You can even sauté foods using chicken stock instead of oil. Flavor foods with lemon juice, balsamic vinegar, and any other nonfat dressings. Use spices and herbs to add lots of flavor.

I'm not a chef, so I don't have a lot of fancy recipes to share, but there are a number of wonderful low-fat cookbooks on the market. Many of the recipes are labor-intensive and might be overly time-consuming (I'd rather see you out getting some aerobic exercise), but if you find the time to cook, and you enjoy it, give one of these a try:

Easy Low-Fat Cooking, by Betty Crocker (Macmillan, $15)
In the Kitchen with Rosie: Oprah's Favorite Recipes, by Rosie Daley (Knopf, $14.95)
Simple and Healthy Cooking, by Jacques Pepin (Rodale Press, $24.95)

Now let's get down to business.

CALORIES: WHAT'S YOUR MAGIC NUMBER ANYWAY?

Earlier I mentioned the three metabolisms. As a reminder, your basal metabolism is what keeps your body running if you just lie in bed twenty-four hours a day and do *nothing*. In general, a woman's basal metabolism burns about 1,200 calories a day, while a man's burns about 1,500. Do those numbers sound familiar? That's because most diets suggest this be the number of calories you consume, so that, with some daily exercise, you will create a caloric deficit, which will cause you to lose fat.

Now I'm going to show you how to calculate the number of calories that *your* body requires each day according to your weight and lean muscle mass (LMM). These numbers are general; your caloric requirements will fluctuate from day to day depending on many factors. For our purposes this will help you to make general guidelines for what you should be eating each day. Here's how to figure out your basal metabolic rate (BMR):

Determine lean muscle mass   Multiply LMM by 16 (kcal)
   (page 144)   _____   _____Total calories

This number is the number of calories that you require to support your current lean muscle mass. If you want to *maintain* your current weight, this is how many calories you should eat each day. If you want to:

Lose body fat aggressively: subtract 500
Lose body fat moderately: subtract 250
Lose body fat very gradually: use BMR
Gain muscle mass: add 500

WARNING: Lowering your caloric intake more than 500 calories will cause you to lose lean muscle mass.

Insert your planned Daily Caloric Consumption_____

Your BMR will change as you progress in the program. As you gain muscle and lose fat, your body will require more calories to function. As you lose body fat, recalculate your caloric needs according to the above formula. Now let's break this equation down even further to determine what substrates or fuels those calories should be coming from.

DAILY REQUIREMENTS MADE SIMPLE

As you have probably noticed, most eating plans are organized by category of food like carbohydrates, proteins, and fats. Then they are further defined by percentage to indicate how much of each category you should have each day. Peak 10 is organized the same way. It is necessary to use percentages so that each individual (with his or her different caloric needs) can be certain he or she is eating a balanced diet. So Peak 10 recommends:

70% of calories from carbohydrates
15% of calories from protein
15% of calories from fat

This is significantly different from the recommendations by the U.S. Department of Agriculture/U.S. Department of Health and Human Services. I recommend less fat, because you're trying to *change* your body, and change will take place faster if you eat less fat. Now let's figure out what that means specifically for you. Here's how to determine your daily percentages, using your Daily Caloric Consumption from the preceding page.

For the number of *carbohydrate* calories you need,
    multiply your Daily Caloric Consumption by .70.   C _____
For the number of *protein* calories you need, multiply
    your Daily Caloric Consumption by .15.   P _____
For the number of *fat* calories you need, multiply your
    Daily Caloric Consumption by .15.   F _____

Let's go through these numbers using an actual person so that you can see how it works. I have a client who has been training hard for six weeks now. At 125 pounds, she is 18 percent body fat. That means that she has 22.5 pounds of fat, so if we subtract 22.5 from 125, we get her lean muscle mass, which is 102.5. Now we multiply 102.5 times 16 (kcal) and come up with 1,640. That is the total number of calories, or energy, that it takes to support her lean muscle mass. If her diet falls more than 500 calories below this, she is in danger of losing lean muscle mass. That will lower her metabolism. So she needs to eat a *minimum* of 1,140 calories per day.

Let's say that she is on one of those starvation diets, and isn't working with weights. She gets down to 120 pounds. You might think that sounds great, but let's look a little deeper and pinch some fat. We have determined that her body fat is now 33 percent. That means she is 80 pounds of LMM. Now we multiply 80 times 16 (kcal) and come up with 1,280. Hey, she's burning fewer calories now—360 per day, to be exact! And guess what: She can't drink those stupid 1,000-calorie-a-day shakes forever, so she's going to put on more weight, and now she's worse off than before she started her diet.

So you see why it is so important to keep exercising and not to starve yourself. It can be broken down to numbers, and the numbers don't lie!

Meal-by-Meal Breakdown of Grams

Now we are going to outline what each meal that you eat during the day will consist of in terms of grams of carbohydrates, protein, and fat. This will make it easier for you to count the grams on the nutrition labels provided on most foods, and use them to gauge how much you should be eating throughout the day. You also might want to purchase a calorie counter to look up some of the foods that don't have labels. There are many available. Just be sure that you get one that gives not only calories but fat grams, protein grams, carbohydrate grams, and sodium if you're watching your salt intake. Once you look something up a couple of times, you will start to remember what it provides and how it fits into your daily intake.

Here's how to fill in your numbers:

Sample Day

From preceding page, take "C," "P," and "F" and fill them in below, then perform the math.

Breakfast

C _____ ×.25= _____ divide by 4= _____ g of carbs
P _____ ×.25= _____ divide by 4= _____ g of protein
F _____ ×.25= _____ divide by 9= _____ g of fat

Morning Snack

C _____ ×.05= _____ divide by 4= _____ g of carbs
P _____ ×.05= _____ divide by 4= _____ g of protein
F _____ ×.05= _____ divide by 9= _____ g of fat

Lunch

C _____ ×.25= _____ divide by 4= _____ g of carbs
P _____ ×.25= _____ divide by 4= _____ g of protein
F _____ ×.25= _____ divide by 9= _____ g of fat

Afternoon Snack

C	_____	×.10=	_____	divide by 4=	_____ g of carbs
P	_____	×.10=	_____	divide by 4=	_____ g of protein
F	_____	×.10=	_____	divide by 9=	_____ g of fat

Dinner

C	_____	×.30=	_____	divide by 4=	_____ g of carbs
P	_____	×.30=	_____	divide by 4=	_____ g of protein
F	_____	×.30=	_____	divide by 9=	_____ g of fat

Late Snack

C	_____	×.05=	_____	divide by 4=	_____ g of carbs
P	_____	×.05=	_____	divide by 4=	_____ g of protein
F	_____	×.05=	_____	divide by 9=	_____ g of fat

The above table calculates the number of grams that you need each day of carbohydrates, protein, and fat, based on your daily caloric requirements. You can see how each meal breaks down according to your daily grams of each as well. Now, let's be realistic: People don't really eat like this, do they? So this is only a guideline for you to base your daily meals upon. If you eat a larger breakfast, then maybe you should make dinner or lunch a little lighter. You can carry grams over from snacks and meals. For example, if you were 10 grams of protein short for breakfast, you need a little extra lean protein at some other point in the day. Don't cheat yourself. The reason I've divided it this way is that I want you to get accustomed to eating smaller meals throughout the day. This is how you will change your body.

To help you continue this pattern of eating through the ten weeks and beyond, I include the table below in your exercise assignments each day. That way you can keep track of your eating patterns more easily. If you do it right, you will improve your body and your health—I guarantee it.

You can practice filling this in now. All you need to do is fill in your projected grams on the left, then write in the foods that you eat on the right, with their estimated grams. This way you can see where you stand at each meal and snack.

All this calorie and gram counting can be time-consuming and sometimes frustrating. But once you do it for a few days, you will start to know what the numbers are, and you'll know what it should feel like. You will know when you are sticking to the program and when you are not.

From preceding table, take gram totals for each meal and snack and fill in on the left. Then fill in grams and foods beside each total.

Breakfast

_____ g of carbs   _____ g of carbs   _____
_____ g of protein _____ g of protein _____
_____ g of fat   _____ g of fat   _____

Morning Snack

_____ g of carbs   _____ g of carbs   _____
_____ g of protein _____ g of protein _____
_____ g of fat   _____ g of fat   _____

Lunch

_____ g of carbs   _____ g of carbs   _____
_____ g of protein _____ g of protein _____
_____ g of fat   _____ g of fat   _____

Afternoon Snack

_____ g of carbs   _____ g of carbs   _____
_____ g of protein _____ g of protein _____
_____ g of fat   _____ g of fat   _____

Dinner

_____ g of carbs   _____ g of carbs   _____
_____ g of protein _____ g of protein _____
_____ g of fat   _____ g of fat   _____

Late Snack

_____ g of carbs   _____ g of carbs   _____
_____ g of protein _____ g of protein _____
_____ g of fat   _____ g of fat   _____

To help you categorize the foods that you eat, following are some examples of the best sources of carbohydrates and proteins, and how to avoid fat.

CARBOHYDRATES

- *Vegetables:* spinach, broccoli, leafy greens, asparagus, cauliflower, brussels sprouts, carrots, celery, peppers, tomatoes, V-8 juice (low sodium), squash, zucchini, green beans, tomato sauce, eggplant, peas, corn, sweet potatoes, potatoes
- *Fruits:* cantaloupe, apples, papaya, strawberries, mango, kiwi, melon, oranges, grapefruit, peaches, plums, grapes, apricots, watermelon, bananas, pears, nectarines, blueberries, raspberries, fruit juices, dried fruits (more calories than fresh fruit)
- *Breads, cereal, rice, and pasta:* whole-wheat bread, grain bread, low-cal bread, pitas, bagels, Wasa bread, English muffins, high-fiber/low-sugar cereals, rice, wild rice, oatmeal, bran, pasta, spinach or tomato pasta.

PROTEIN

- *Dairy:* skim milk, nonfat yogurt, nonfat cottage cheese, nonfat sour cream, nonfat cheese slices, egg whites, Egg Beaters
- *Meat, poultry, fish:* fresh fish fillet, tuna or salmon steaks, shrimp, scallops, clams, oysters, white-meat chicken or turkey, tuna packed in water
- *Legumes (beans):* lentils, cannellini beans, kidney beans, chickpeas, white beans, black beans, black-eyed peas, bean sprouts, split green peas, split yellow peas, lima beans, light tofu.

AVOID FATS

You probably already know which foods are high in fat, and that you should avoid them. It might be difficult for you to stop eating fatty foods "cold turkey," though. Doing something too abruptly will only set you up for failure. To stay on track, begin by reducing your fat intake *gradually*. Switch from whole milk to 2 percent, to 1 percent, then to skim. Sprinkle a little cheese on top of foods rather than baking it throughout. Try making "home fries" by spraying shoestring potatoes lightly with Pam spray and baking them rather than frying. If you *have* to have cream cheese, and don't like the fat-free variety, then spread it *thinly* rather than globbing it on a bagel. These little changes will yield big results over time.

Sources of fat include whole milk, yogurt, or other whole dairy products, red meat, pork, processed meats (bacon, corned beef, hot dogs, pastrami, salami, sausages), fried foods (this includes fried potatoes, fried chicken, fried shrimp, and fried vegetables), gravy, skin on poultry or fish, egg yolks, cheese, oils, dressings, coconut, avocado, nuts, seeds, and olives.

GROCERY LIST

TOMATOES
SWEET POTATOES
ROMAINE LETTUCE
CARROTS
CELERY
EGGPLANT
MUSHROOMS
GREEN AND RED PEPPERS
BRUSSELS SPROUTS
BEAN SPROUTS
MACINTOSH APPLES
BANANAS
PEARS
CANTALOUPE
STRAWBERRIES
ORANGE JUICE
SKIM OR 1% MILK
NONFAT SUGAR-FREE YOGURT
NONFAT PLAIN YOGURT
NONFAT COTTAGE CHEESE
FAT-FREE SOUR CREAM
FAT-FREE CHEESE SLICES
THINLY SLICED FRESH TURKEY
CANNED WHITE TUNA PACKED IN WATER (check fat content, they vary)
DRIED LENTILS OR SPLIT PEAS
WHOLE CHICKEN FOR ROASTING
CANNELLINI BEANS
FRESH TUNA STEAKS
LO-CAL WHOLE-WHEAT BREAD
WHOLE-WHEAT LINGUINI
BROWN RICE
COUSCOUS
WASA CRISPBREAD CRACKERS
PAM COOKING SPRAY

CREATING A DEFICIT

There is something else that we can use besides diet to improve our fitness level: We can be *active* people. You will move in play and at work. Your body will expend additional calories over and above the basal metabolic needs that you've determined above. Just as our food has caloric values, so do the activities we partake in. So we use more than 1,200 or 1,500 calories every day. However, most of us consume a much greater number of calories than we expend. In fact, occasionally we might eat 1,200 calories in *one* meal. So if one of your goals is to reduce body fat, the trick is to reduce the intake while increasing the expenditures and *voilà!* You have less fat to carry around.

Your additional daily expenditures in the form of exercise will go hand in hand with your diet to boost fat loss. *You need to use 3,600 calories to lose one pound of body fat.* This number is the same for everyone. If you jog or walk each day enough to burn 600 calories, and reduce your consumption to 400 calories under your BMR, then you will be creating a deficit of 1,000 calories per day and will lose a pound of fat every three and a half days. This is how you should design your eating plan. You need to calculate your rate of weight loss by creating a caloric deficit through exercise and a personalized eating plan.

Nanny Besio's Pasta e Fagioli

3 quick sprays olive oil cooking spray
1 tsp. chopped garlic
1 28-oz. can whole chopped tomatoes, drained
5 leaves fresh basil, minced
¾ lb. tubettini or tubetti pasta
1 19-oz. can cannellini beans
2 tsp. balsamic vinegar
Salt and pepper to taste
1 tbs. Parmesan cheese

Put on a large pot of lightly salted water to boil for the pasta. Coat saucepan lightly with olive oil spray and sauté garlic until lightly browned. Add chopped tomatoes and fresh basil and simmer for 30 minutes. Put pasta on to boil. Add cannellini beans and vinegar to saucepan. Let cook, but don't overstir or you'll crush the beans. Drain pasta, add to saucepan, and toss together (you can toss it in a separate bowl if it doesn't fit). Serve a portion the size of your fist and sprinkle lightly with Parmesan. (Of course, Nanny Besio would never give you a portion that small, but we have to start changing some things, don't we?)

Serving size: 1½ cups (about 315 calories). 58g of carbohydrate, 14g of protein, 2g of fat

BEDTIME SNACK

Okay, it's time for your last snack of the day. What should it be? Ice cream? No, too much fat and you've learned about fat. Jelly beans? No, too much sugar and you've learned about sugar. Alcohol? No, a waste of calories, and besides, contrary to popular belief, you'll sleep better without it. Give up? Okay. Now's the perfect time for a frozen banana, or a sorbet, and some chamomile tea. Or you could make a Health Shake.

A Cool Health Shake

1 8-oz. container nonfat sugar-free banana-strawberry yogurt
1 ripe banana
½ cup skim milk
1 tbs. vanilla extract
½ cup ice
1 packet artificial sweetener

Combine all ingredients in a blender and blend to desired consistency.

If you're out on the town, you can top off your meal with one of those great high-maintenance coffee drinks. A little something to end the day, without straying from your plan. Decaf cappuccino with skim milk and Equal is my personal favorite. Just make sure that you're reasonable and moderate and you'll be sticking to the program. Speaking of which, I have some tips that might help you.

STICKING TO THE PLAN

Most important, don't torture yourself if you eat something that you shouldn't have, or if you eat too much of something, or if you accidentally go out and drink a couple of martinis with five olives each, or if you do all those things in one night. An occasional straying from your plan, a slice of birthday cake here and there, should be no excuse to stop Peak 10. The point is that you need to be really disciplined for ten weeks so that you can learn what it takes to go on and live a balanced lifestyle after that. And I'm glad to say that a balanced lifestyle does include some unhealthful foods every so often.

Be aware of how your eating will affect your body, and balance it with every other aspect of your life. Who knows, you might want to walk an extra half hour someday (and I hope that you do!). It all gets calculated into the equation.

PEAK 10 TIPS FOR HEALTHFUL EATING

- *Become more aware of the foods you eat.* You will use your Dietary Recall, and then your caloric breakdown counter, to help you monitor your eating habits.
- *Eat a low-fat diet.* The bulk of your diet should consist of carbohydrates. Fruits and vegetables are a great source of this important nutrient, as are potatoes, breads, and cereals.
- *Drink plenty of water.* The average adult needs six to eight 8-ounce glasses a day to maintain general good health. Additionally, you should drink about 4 ounces of water for every fifteen minutes that you exercise.
- *Eat three to five servings of vegetables per day.* The key is to avoid butter or high-fat sauces. Vinegar, Worcestershire sauce, and mustard can all be used to add flavor to vegetables without adding fat.
- *Eat two to four servings of fruit per day.* Fruit makes a great, healthful snack, and it's easy to take on the run.
- *Avoid foods that are high in sugar.* Even fat-free and low-fat desserts and snacks are often very high in calories, and the sugar in these foods is easily converted to fat.
- *Choose foods that are high in fiber.* Fruits, vegetables, and high-fiber cereals are great sources.

- *Keep track of the* amount *of food you eat.* Choosing low-fat foods is important, but it is possible to eat too much of almost *any* kind of food. Reading labels on food containers will help you determine appropriate portion sizes.
- *Be sure to eat three meals a day.* Breakfast is especially important. But skipping any meal will deprive you of the energy and nutrients you need to function well. What's more, if you skip meals, you're more likely to overindulge when you do sit down to eat. Don't forget your healthy snacks!
- *Think in terms of moderation, not deprivation.* There's no need to completely deprive yourself of the foods you love. But it is extremely important to eat a well-balanced diet to avoid consuming more calories than you burn.

PEAK 10 MEAL PLAN MADE EASY

If you don't have the time to spend planning elaborate healthy meals, or you still aren't sure what you should be eating, we've made it simple for you. Below are eleven sample days of meals, grouped by breakfast, lunch, dinner, and snacks. Use the daily calorie intake that you calculated for yourself on page 66, and put together some meals from the selections below that add up to your calorie plan. You can decrease the portion size of something in the meal if you want to lower the calories, or increase the quantity to raise the caloric value. Be certain to keep a good balance of protein to carbohydrates and fat.

Following these sample meals will help you see exactly how to eat to be lean and fit.

BREAKFAST
1 cup yogurt, nonfat
½ medium cantaloupe
calories: 205

1 piece (6″ diam.) pita, whole wheat

Omelet:

3 fl. ounces Egg Beaters
½ cup mushrooms, raw
½ medium pepper, raw
½ medium onion, raw
½ cup spinach, raw
1 slice tomato
    calories: 211

—————

Egg white omelet:

5 large egg whites
½ cup mushrooms, raw
½ medium pepper, raw
4 slices tomato
1 piece (6″ diam.) pita, whole wheat
¼ medium cantaloupe
    calories: 241

—————

4 large egg whites
1 piece (6″ diam.) pita, whole wheat
1 cup yogurt, nonfat
    calories: 254

—————

4 fl. ounces Egg Beaters
1 piece corn tortilla
1 medium banana
    calories: 276

—————

¼ medium honeydew melon
1 piece (4″ diam.) pita, whole wheat
½ cup cottage cheese, nonfat
    calories: 280

—————

1 medium bagel, whole wheat
1 medium banana
    calories: 290

—————

½ cup Oat Bran hot cereal
4 dates, dried
1 tablespoon honey
   calories: 292

------

1 cup yogurt, nonfat
¼ cup raisins
1 slice seven grain bread
1 tablespoon fruit spread, any flavor
   calories: 315

------

2 ounces oatmeal hot cereal without salt
1 medium banana
   calories: 325

------

2 ounces shredded wheat with bran
¼ cup raisins
1 cup milk, skim
   calories: 414

LUNCH

½ medium cantaloupe
½ cup cottage cheese, nonfat
1 piece (4″ diam.) pita, whole wheat
   calories: 264

------

3 ounces tuna, canned, in water
1 piece (6″ diam.) pita, whole wheat
1 tablespoon vinegar
1 cup lettuce
1 medium apple
   calories: 300

------

2 cups lettuce
4 ounces shrimp, broiled
1 piece (4″ diam.) pita, whole wheat
4 slices tomato
1 medium orange
   calories: 311

------

1 cup bean soup, low sodium, no fat
½ cup brown rice, cooked
1 cup lettuce
4 slices tomato
½ cup cucumber, raw
2 medium kiwi
  calories: 361

————

1 piece (6″ diam.) pita, whole wheat
1 tablespoon mustard
1 medium tomato, raw
1 cup lettuce
2 ounces turkey light, without skin
1 medium banana
  calories: 379

————

1 medium roll, wheat
1 tablespoon mustard
4 slices tomato, raw
4 ounces chicken breast, without skin
1 medium apple
  calories: 384

————

1 medium potato, baked with skin
½ cup cottage cheese, nonfat
½ cup cucumber, raw
4 slices tomato, raw
1 medium apple
  calories: 414

————

2 cups salad, tossed
1 tablespoon vinegar
2 slices seven grain bread
4 ounces tuna, canned, in water
4 slices tomato, raw
1 medium apple
  calories: 424

————

1 medium bagel, whole wheat
3 ounces turkey light, without skin
1 cup lettuce
1 tablespoon mustard
2 medium figs, dried
   calories: 445

---

1 cup pasta, cooked
½ cup carrots, cooked
1 medium tomato, raw
½ cup cucumber, raw
3 ounces tuna, canned, in water
1 medium apple
   calories: 473

---

1 cup brown rice, cooked
½ cup broccoli, cooked
1 tablespoon vinegar
¾ cup garbanzo beans, cooked
1 medium apple
   calories: 538

DINNER

4 ounces chicken breast, without skin
2 pieces corn tortillas
4 tablespoons salsa
2 cups lettuce
   calories: 364

---

1 cup wild rice, cooked
½ cup garbanzo beans, canned
½ cup spinach, cooked
½ cup zucchini, cooked
2 tablespoons salsa
   calories: 367

1 cup salad, tossed
1 cup pasta, cooked
½ cup tomato sauce
½ cup asparagus, cooked
½ cup broccoli, cooked
   calories: 370
   ———————

1 cup lettuce
5 ounces red snapper, broiled
½ cup brown rice, cooked
½ cup green beans, cooked
½ cup broccoli, cooked
½ medium grapefruit
   calories: 394
   ———————

5 ounces chicken breast, without skin
1 cup lettuce
1 tablespoon vinegar
½ medium potato, baked with skin
1 cup asparagus, cooked
2 dates, dried
   calories: 450
   ———————

5 ounces salmon, broiled
½ medium sweet potato
1 cup spinach, cooked
½ cup peas, cooked
1 medium nectarine
   calories: 463
   ———————

1 cup lettuce
5 fl. ounces Egg Beaters
1 cup asparagus, cooked
1 medium potato, baked with skin
1 medium banana
   calories: 470
   ———————

5 ounces turkey light, without skin
½ cup brown rice, cooked
½ cup broccoli, cooked
1 cup carrots, cooked
1 medium orange
  calories: 486

———————

1 cup pasta, cooked
½ cup tomato sauce
1 cup broccoli, cooked
1 medium artichoke, cooked
½ cup kidney beans, canned
  calories: 505

———————

8 ounces shrimp, broiled
2 cups lettuce
1 medium artichoke, cooked
½ medium potato, baked with skin
1 medium apple
  calories: 509

———————

1 medium potato, baked with skin
½ cup zucchini, cooked
½ cup cauliflower, cooked
¼ cup cottage cheese, nonfat
½ cup baked beans, plain
1 medium pear
  calories: 510

SNACKS

1 medium fig, dried
2 medium apricots
  calories: 82

———————

½ medium cantaloupe
  calories: 94

———————

2 pieces Wasa fiber plus
1 tablespoon fruit spread, any flavor
½ medium grapefruit
  calories: 150

---

1 medium banana
2 dates, dried
  calories: 151

---

1 medium apple
1 cup yogurt, nonfat
  calories: 181

---

1 medium banana
½ cup frozen yogurt, nonfat
  calories: 195

---

1 medium pear
1 cup yogurt, fruit, nonfat
  calories: 198

---

1 cup yogurt, nonfat
1 medium banana
  calories: 205

---

1 cup yogurt, nonfat
2 dates, dried
1 medium apple
  calories: 227

---

2 medium figs, dried
½ medium cantaloupe
1 cup yogurt, fruit, nonfat
  calories: 243

---

1 cup yogurt, nonfat
1 medium apple
15 grapes
  calories: 253

ANNE'S STORY

I decided to try Peak 10 because I had put on a lot of weight after having a heart attack. I stayed in the hospital for a while, and had to quit smoking (which I should have done a long time ago!), both of which led to my gaining weight. I had a terrible time getting rid of the weight because I believed that I wasn't eating very much.

I was friends with one of Chris's trainers and she told me to keep a food diary, but I thought I had better things to do back then. Finally I realized that I had a choice: I could try the program or still be fat.

The first step for me was having Chris give me a list of what to eat. I wanted him to show me what one day on Peak 10 would be like. With the food and shopping lists I was able to manipulate my eating schedule. In all honesty, I was afraid to do this because you eat every couple of hours—I thought I'd put on weight. I felt like I was eating constantly. On Peak 10 you eat throughout the day.

Chris is wonderful because he is very realistic about keeping everything in moderation. I followed the program to the letter during the day, but because I cooked dinner for a bunch of people, that was the one meal

Anne Age: 39 Height: 5'7"	*Start*	*Finish*
MEASUREMENTS		
Neck	13	12.25
Shoulders	41	39.5
Chest	38.5	36.5
Waist	35.5	32
Hips	43	40.25
Rt. Thigh	25.75	23.5
Rt. Calf	15.75	15
Rt. Upper Arm	11.75	11
Rt. Forearm	10.5	10
Weight	170	149
% Fat	36.8/36.8	25.5/24.9
TOTAL INCHES	234.75	220
Inches lost 14.75		

I didn't change. I made sure I had a reasonable portion of pasta with salad. It was very much a normal dinner, although I wouldn't eat seconds. I wasn't hungry ever. The best part was that no one told me I was doing it wrong. Chris just gave me suggestions to make the meal I wanted to eat a little healthier.

I walked at least a half hour every day and tried to do an hour of walking at least three times a week. Then, after quite a few weeks I started to take my bike out because I felt more energetic and wanted to push a little more. So I wasn't killing myself with the exercise, although every other morning I did the weight thing. I did the upper body weights one day and the lower body another. On the weekends I tried to do a little bit more. I didn't feel restricted because of my heart attack and my exercise program wasn't restricted by my doctor. Chris knew my health history and tailored my program accordingly.

After about three or four weeks into the program I noticed that my shorts felt looser . . . nothing major, but they weren't snug. Then, very shortly after that, the weight just flew off me. It was the weirdest thing. My whole body changed. It took a while and then once I noticed the difference, I was really inspired. Toward the end of the ten weeks, I put on a pair of jeans that I hadn't worn in a while (because by then I had started to slip into things that were in the back of my closet) and they weren't snug. I didn't realize how big they were until I passed by a mirror and saw the rear end of the pants sticking out about three inches. I immediately went shopping and found out that I had lost two sizes. It was terribly exciting. At the beginning of Peak 10, I was heading toward 180 pounds after being a size eight or ten my whole life—and I was back into a size ten!

Five months later I haven't put the weight back on—that's what's amazing to me. I'm not officially on Peak 10 anymore, but I am very aware of what I eat. It was such a slow weight loss that it allowed me to really change my lifestyle. My body right now feels like it did ten years ago when I was thirty. I don't feel like I did when I was twenty, but I feel great that I look like this at forty.

If I get hungry my snack is instant oatmeal. It gives me something hot to eat. I put Polaner All-fruit on it. And these days I always have an apple or four hard-boiled eggs in my bag. And I'm never far from some tuna fish and carrots. People don't like to plan what they're going to eat, but if you make room to think ahead, then you can really keep the weight off.

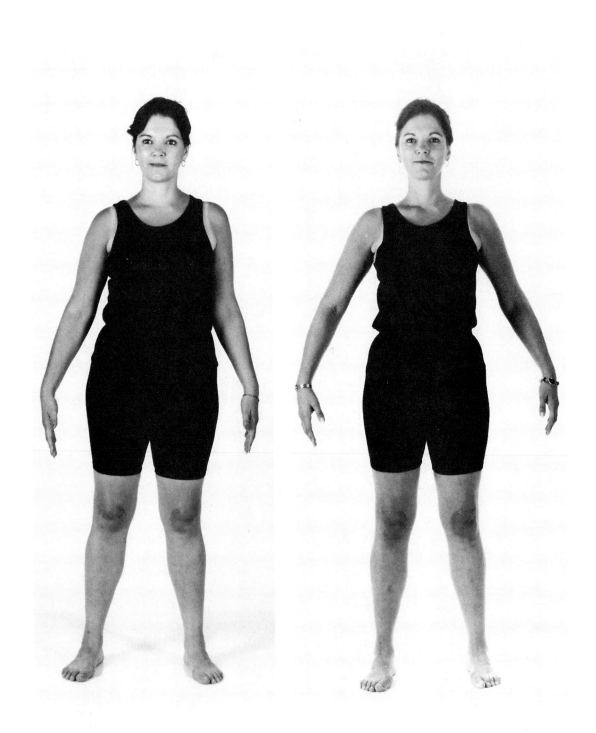

Ten weeks is such a short period of time to have an enormous result. In ten weeks you can change your whole life or you can still be complaining. I'm very proud of my pictures. I'm really proud of what happened to me and what I was able to do in ten weeks because I made a commitment.

5

Building a Fat-Burning Machine

When I mention the word *aerobic,* most people think of a group of people jumping around to loud music, shaking sweat on each other. Well, the truth is we all do lots of things that are aerobic, some without even realizing it. In terms of exercise, aerobic simply means conditioning the heart and lungs by means of increased oxygen intake. Just as you can't light a match in space, you can't burn fat without oxygen. A good session of nonstop vacuuming, a slow climb up a long flight of stairs, and a walk around the shopping mall are all aerobic activities that will increase your oxygen intake.

In this chapter, we will take you through the steps to determine the intensity at which you should be training aerobically to burn the most amount of stored fat. Along with burning fat, we will also use aerobic training to strengthen and condition your cardiovascular system. We will use a combination of different training techniques to optimize your Peak 10 results.

HOW DO WE DO IT?

In order to increase your heart and respiratory rates, you've got to move. When you move, your body's physiology changes. As your heartbeat quickens, you feel a warm tingly feeling throughout your body. Over time, your heart, being the most important muscle in your body, gets stronger from the added activity. You are exercising.

Like resistance weight training, aerobic conditioning is controlled stress. Your body will gradually adapt to aerobic activity when given in the proper doses (we will determine your personal Target Training Zone and Optimum Fat Utilization Zone). Over time, with graduated progression, your heart is able to pump more blood more easily. You don't need to be a world-class athlete to appreciate the benefits of a strong heart and lungs. By moving, you are getting ready to ascend to the peak, and I'm coming with you.

CHOOSE TO MOVE

You can move in many ways. It's all up to you. Do you like to walk, run, swim, or hike? Does cycling do it for you? Whatever activity you enjoy and find fun, do it. As long as you can do it at a steady pace and the activity increases your heart rate, you are conditioning your cardiovascular system and burning fat. When it comes to burning fat, we need to perform aerobic activities that allow control over our rate of exertion, or intensity.

There are a few activities that I don't recommend for maximum fat burning:

Racket sports. They tend to be stop-and-go.
Golf. Great fun, but it's not terribly active.
Weight lifting. This is anaerobic, meaning without oxygen.
Bowling. Too much sitting and beer.
Any activity that you find difficult or dangerous (for example, in-line skating if you aren't good at it, or downhill skiing).

These are all fun activities. I'm not recommending that you don't do them, but they simply aren't the best way to improve your fat-burning ability. Enjoy these activities on your "off time" for fun and relaxation.

The exercises that I do recommend to get your heart working are walking, running, stair climbing, biking, hiking, swimming, rowing— any activity that allows you complete control over the intensity. You need to be able to speed up and slow down to maintain your rates. But before you get started, you need to know what intensity or intensities you should be training at to get the job done. Let me explain.

DETERMINING YOUR TRAINING ZONES

To maximize your results, aerobic training and cardio conditioning need to be broken down into four categories: warm-up, OFUZ (Optimum Fat Utilization Zone), cardio conditioning training zone, and cool-down.

To determine these zones, we first need to determine your resting pulse. Sit down in a relaxed and comfortable position. Locate your pulse, either at the base of your wrist, using your index and middle fingers, or at the side of your neck, using the same two fingers. Be sure not to press too hard; doing so can artificially lower your heart rate.

To assure a more accurate reading, try to sit quietly for a few minutes before taking your pulse. Start a stopwatch or monitor the second hand of a clock and count your pulse for fifteen seconds. Multiply this number by 4. This is your resting heart rate. For example, if you counted sixteen beats, $16 \times 4 = 64$ beats per minute.

Resting heart rate: _____

To determine your estimated maximum heart rate, subtract your age from 220. For example:

$$220 - 35 \text{ (your age)} = 185$$

Estimated maximum heart rate: _____

To determine your Target Training Zone, we will establish boundaries that will enable us to pinpoint the levels of intensity for a specific goal.

The age-adjusted low end of your training zone is determined by first subtracting your resting heart rate from your estimated maximum heart rate. For example:

185 (estimated maximum heart rate) − 64 (resting heart rate) = 121

Age-adjusted maximum heart rate: _____

Using your resting heart rate personalizes this zone for you. Now, multiply your age-adjusted maximum heart rate by 55 percent (.55) and add to that number your resting heart rate to determine the low end of your target training zone. For example:

$$121 \times .55 - 64 = 131$$

Low end of Target Training Zone: _____

This is the low end of your Target Training Zone. In other words, if your heart is beating 131 beats per minute, you are exercising very moder-

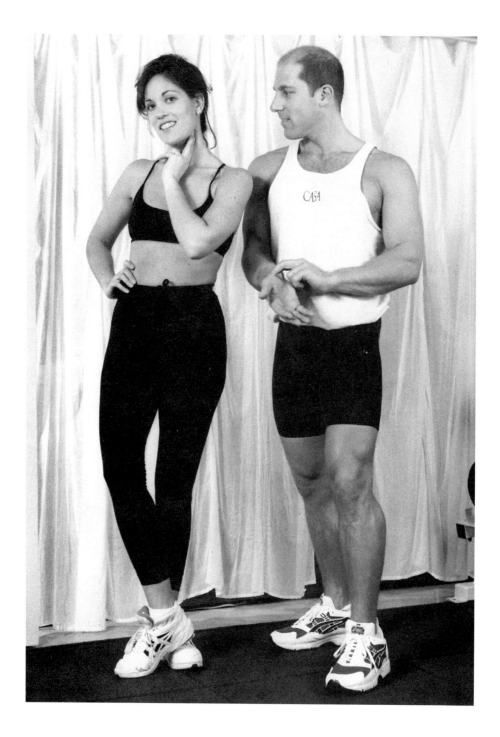

ately. Your heart is pumping more than it does at rest, but it's not to the point of overexertion.

To find the high end of your Target Training Zone, multiply your age-adjusted maximum heart rate by 90 percent (.90) and then once again add your resting heart rate. For example:

$$121 \times .90 + 64 = 173$$

High end of Target Training Zone _____

IMPORTANT: The numbers that you've just calculated will change as your fitness level improves. Retest yourself every two weeks to be sure that you are working at the best pace for you.

Now that you've established your resting heart rate along with your Target Training Zone, you need to warm up before you can even consider training in this zone.

THE WARM-UP

The warm-up occurs between your resting heart rate and the low end of your Target Training Zone. Warming up serves a couple of purposes. As you gradually increase your heart rate from resting to the lower level of your target zone, your body temperature increases and your muscles become more flexible, thereby reducing your risk of injury. Warming up gradually also encourages your body to continue to use fat as a major fuel source as the intensity increases. During the warm-up you should check your pulse a few times to be sure you're pushing yourself enough—but not too much.

Let's say you decide to go for a run. Once out of your front door, you try to get right into a groove, but your body starts to sputter halfway down the block. You feel a burn in your muscles and you're sucking wind. This run that came to a sudden stop burned mostly sugar that is stored in your muscles, but it didn't use very much fat from the major fuel reserves in your hips, waist, and thighs.

Because you didn't allow your body enough time to call on its fat stores for energy by warming up, it went into a "fight or flight" response. There are built-in survival mechanisms that allow us to defend ourselves or get away from trouble quickly through energy stored directly in our muscles. This is the energy that your body uses when it doesn't have time to process your fat stores for energy. Unfortunately, it's not enough juice to get very far.

Because of the way that we use energy, we need to warm up slowly and gradually allow our body time to access our fat stores and convert them to energy. So if fat reduction is a goal, warming up will be a critical part of your Peak 10 program.

Now let's use what you just learned about your aerobic training zone to work more efficiently and burn more fat. This time you warm up for ten minutes, then walk briskly while keeping your heart rate within your zone for thirty minutes, then you cool down.

During your exercise you used some of the stored fat from your body while safely keeping your sugar levels steady. You didn't get too tired or feel sluggish. In fact, you still feel kind of energized at the end of the day.

When your body needs energy immediately—for example, if you run quickly without warming up—it will use the quickest fuel available. And that's always a sugar. Because you called on your muscles to move so quickly, your body went into overdrive and bypassed the stored fat.

However, when you exercised in your Target Training Zone, your body never went into fight-or-flight mode. Instead, because you started out slowly, your body thought, "Well, I'm safe here. It looks like I have time to break down these fat cells for energy." So it provided you with a steady source of fat to burn.

Maximize all of your Peak 10 workouts. Before aerobic activity, always warm up for five to ten minutes, depending on how long you will be training. Giving yourself that time to pick up the pace allows your body to burn stored fat for longer, more productive workouts. Soon you'll get used to the way your body feels when it's in the proper warm-up zone, and you won't have to monitor your pulse.

OFUZ

We've narrowed down your training zone based on your resting heart rate and age. Now I want to further pinpoint the zone that I refer to as your Optimum Fat Utilization Zone, or OFUZ. Your OFUZ—your fat-burning zone—strikes the balance between duration and intensity that allows your body to burn the most fat calories. This zone is directly below the "Anaerobic Threshold," which can be pinpointed by using the "Talk Test." When you are exercising and reach the point where you can no longer talk comfortably, or carry a tune, you are no longer delivering sufficient oxygen to your cells and are nearing your Anaerobic Threshold. When our focus is on losing body fat, we don't want to push ourselves above our Anaerobic Threshold. Not getting enough oxygen will only diminish our body's ability to burn fat.

When you reach your anaerobic threshold, continue exercising steadily as you take your pulse, and record this number. This is the number that you use as the high end of your OFUZ. As you become more fit, this number will increase, so remember to continuously practice the Talk Test and make the appropriate adjustments.

Once you've approximated your Anaerobic Threshold, find your OFUZ by taking that number and subtracting 10. This 10-beat range is your OFUZ.

OFUZ _____

It's important to remember that fat needs oxygen to burn. "Aerobic" is just shorthand for "exercise with oxygen." You'll give your body the oxygen it needs to burn the proper proportions of fat and sugar when you're working at the right pace.

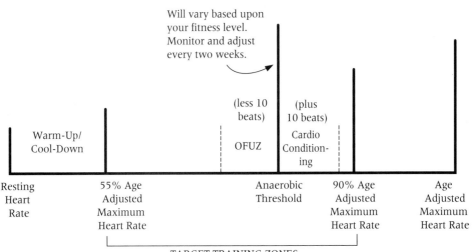

CARDIO CONDITIONING

When it comes to training and conditioning your cardiovascular system for maximum performance, you will need to turn up the intensity. I have set aside training days in your program to help strengthen and boost your cardiac output, that is, the amount of blood circulated by your heart each minute. These days are labeled "Cardio Conditioning" and always include a warm-up and cool-down like any other aerobic activity. Refer to the chart on page 94. As the chart indicates, your cardio conditioning zone will require you to raise your heart rate to your anaerobic threshold (when you can no longer talk comfortably) and above—between one and ten beats higher, depending on your fitness level.

Even though your cardiovascular system benefits from any type of aerobic activity, taking the intensity to a higher level for a short time will help to stress your heart, thereby strengthening it. If you've just started exercising, keep your cardiac conditioning level closer to your anaerobic threshold. As always, listen to your body and don't push yourself too hard. Allow ample cool-down time (that means keep moving at a slower pace until your heart rate is below 100 bpm).

GETTING STARTED

What will your workout feel like?

Well, Peak 10—and whatever exercise you choose to do—will always be fun, exciting, sometimes challenging, and it should get results. Whatever activity you choose to do, just be sure that it's something you enjoy, and your training zones will be effective.

START OUT WALKING

If you're new to exercise and aren't sure what you like, try walking. It's easy and effective. How good is walking for you? Add a two-mile workout to your life each day and you decrease your risk of heart disease by 25 percent or more, says one study done by Reebok. In another piece of research, published in the *Journal of the American Medical Association,* December 1991, and conducted at the Institute for Aerobics Research,

102 previously sedentary women in their twenties and thirties walked five days a week at all different speeds. After six months all the groups had lowered their cholesterol and their body fat. They also increased their VO2 max., or aerobic capacity. That means their hearts pumped stronger and better (the groups who walked the fastest experienced the greatest benefits).

After a half hour of walking at a brisk pace you should be breathing a little heavier. Test your Anaerobic Threshold by singing a song to yourself. If you can't sing and are huffing and puffing—then you've reached your Anaerobic Threshold. Or maybe you're like my father-in-law, who never *could* sing, and you should try *talking*. Anyway, we want to do our walking close to this point, but not above it. Slow down a little bit. You should feel an intense workout, but not a stressful one.

Try to keep your level steady for as long as possible. That doesn't mean you have to walk at this pace forever. It just means you should play off the numbers. Eventually you'll know where your heart rate should be and you won't have to check it. You'll be able to slow down based on the feeling you want to achieve.

What does it feel like when your body uses fat as a major source of fuel? It should feel refreshing and exhilarating, not exhausting. No burning and no heavy breathing.

This is your personal aerobic training zone. It should become your best exercise friend, as well as the trainer you would pay $100 an hour for. It allows you to get feedback and information about how your body is doing through your workout. It's just like having someone tell you to slow down or to speed up or that the pace you're walking at is exactly where you want to be.

If you are already exercising regularly, and you've advanced past the walking stage, that's great. I want you to follow your heart rate just like all the other Peakies. What I have found is that some people actually train with their heart rate too high, which doesn't allow them to burn as much fat as they could. So if you're already training regularly, be sure to monitor your heart rate and stay in your OFUZ.

ACTIVITIES BEYOND WALKING

Although walking is a great way to start out the program, because you can control your heart rate, it can get boring for some. As you progress, your body may adapt to the exercise and raising your heart rate may become more difficult. When this happens, increase your speed by walking faster, jogging, walking on an incline, or stair climbing to help raise your heart to the appropriate training level. Taking a friend along can help pass the time more quickly, but if that doesn't work for you, try some new forms of aerobic exercise.

The best aerobic exercise comes from activities that use your major muscle groups, which are those in your butt and legs (quadriceps, gluteals and hamstrings). Muscles expend the majority of energy in our bodies, so the larger the muscle, the more energy it will need to contract and move your limbs. That is why walking, hiking, running, and biking have always been great ways for people to burn body fat. However, other activities such as swimming, rowing, and the upper-body ergometer are effective for people who have knee problems or limited use of the lower body, and can help you get great Peak 10 results as well. Riding a bike, stationary or standard, is a fine alternative if you have ankle or foot problems, or if you just get bored with walking.

The key is to do what works best for you. If you have trouble keeping yourself motivated, you might want to take an aerobics class that you know you'll stick with for the whole hour. To keep herself motivated, my wife likes to run half of her distance in one direction away from home and then turn around and run back. This way she can't stop and shorten her run if she loses motivation, because she still has to get all the way back home, so even if she walks she's still covering the same distance. It is easier to quit early if you're doing a track. If you need to find ways to "trick" yourself into going a little further, that's fine. Just keep yourself motivated.

Some adventurous Peakies might choose to in-line skate or ice-skate. These are great forms of exercise provided you are proficient and practice all the proper safety precautions. And if weather and location permit, a power walk on the beach, some canoeing, mountain biking, and stair climbing are all great aerobic activities. And if you're superadvanced, you can try jumping rope: As long as you keep your heart rate in your OFUZ, the sky's the limit!

If you've tried a lot of these exercises, but still want more variety, try combining two or three activities in a day. This will keep you too busy to get bored. You could do a mini-triathlon by swimming, biking, and running in one day. Or you could create your own triathlon of in-line skating, biking, and canoeing. Do whatever it takes to keep yourself interested, just as long as you don't have too much downtime between activities. If you need to space things out, you'll need to warm up separately each time. And try to keep the core up to at least ten minutes each.

As you can probably tell, I encourage people to get outdoors, but if that's not possible, there are plenty of indoor activities to try, including aerobic videotapes like my Peak 10 video series, the stationary bike, the treadmill, climbing stairs (or stair climbers), or jumping rope, which also travels well.

Speaking of traveling, don't let a trip derail you from your Peak 10 program. Plan to work out where you go by locating a hotel with a fitness club in advance, or a local track or gym near someone you're staying with. You *can* stick with the program on the road. It takes extra effort, but it will pay off in the long run.

Whenever you elevate your heart rate through exercise, it is imperative that you cool down before you stop. Stopping exercise too abruptly can cause blood to pool in your lower body, resulting in lightheadedness or fainting.

To avoid this, complete every exercise session with a less intense activity, such as walking, until your heart rate is below 100 beats per minute. This will allow your body to normalize gradually.

LISTENING TO YOUR BODY

Because this program is new to you, give your body a couple of weeks to become accustomed to it. We've got ten weeks, and remember, each week is building on the one that came before.

Now, before you start, please remember that you have to listen to your body with a sympathetic ear, and speak to it with a kind and inspirational voice. What are your feet, shins, knees, and hips saying? Do we need to pull back a little or speed it up?

Smoking, dehydration, or a cold can affect your heart rate. If it seems high or if you get winded very quickly, slow down and check with your doctor. Most people, though, are perfectly safe walking. Eventually you'll get used to the feelings and be able to work yourself a little harder.

Your body is designed by nature to be comfortable at all times. It adjusts physiologically to make room for changes. We have a mechanism within us called homeostasis that allows us to adapt slowly to new states of being. Your body will take care of you and become comfortable with the slow, gradual changes we ask it to make. But if we rush it and ask too much of ourselves, then our body often breaks down and improvement is limited.

If you want to get leaner and you want to get stronger, just turn it up a little bit more than what you would normally do. You'll get comfortable at that level and it will be time to push it again. Before you know it, you'll be burning fat and changing the way you look and feel. Gradual progress guarantees long-term success.

How long should you work out? Five to ten minutes is key for the warm-up and fat mobilization. Then turn up the intensity. Whether cardio conditioning or fat burning, stay in the appropriate zone on the assigned days. In chapters 8, 9, and 10 I've established progressive training durations for the aerobic components. Try to make these your goals. If you're *less* fit, shoot for a duration that is more comfortable for you . . . don't worry, you'll improve. If you're *more* fit, try to challenge yourself by pushing it to the limit. And be smart about it. I want you around for the whole ten weeks. In fact, I want you to exercise even past these ten weeks, so it might mean walking for twenty minutes the first week, then thirty minutes the second week, and maybe increasing to one hour at the end of your first Peak 10 program.

The only way for you to succeed is for you to be comfortable and enjoy yourself. You're moving, you're feeling good, and this isn't painful. You'll get up tomorrow morning and do it again.

I'd like to tell you one of my favorite stories. It's about Milo the Greek, a guy with a cow in his backyard. At first the cow was just a little calf that weighed a hundred pounds. Every day Milo would go outside and pick the calf up. The calf would gain some weight every week or so, but every week Milo would keep picking him up. At the end of one year the cow weighed a ton and Milo could still lift him, because his body had adapted to the stress gradually.

Milo trained intelligently and so can you. (Just stay away from those *bulls*!)

CHARLENE'S STORY

I was very successful on Peak 10. My body fat went from 36.5% to 29.6%, but more importantly, even after four months without officially being on the program, I've changed a lot of my habits.

I've dieted a zillion different times, and when I started Peak 10 I was

Charlene
Age: 27
Height: 5'7"

MEASUREMENTS	Start	Finish
Neck	13.75	13.25
Shoulders	39.75	37
Chest	38	36
Waist	31	28.5
Hips	42.75	40
Rt. Thigh	26.75	23
Rt. Calf	16	15.5
Rt. Upper Arm	11.5	10.25
Rt. Forearm	10.25	10
Weight	173	159
% Fat	36.3/34.9	29.6/30.2
TOTAL INCHES	229.75	213.5

Inches lost: 16.25

heavier than I'd ever been, but Chris never said, "Don't eat." He was always saying "Eat, eat. Have fruit. Have this. Have that." So he made changing my habits easy. I've noticed a real change in my metabolism. Before I would diet and *boom* the weight would come back again.

Peak 10 wasn't hard and I didn't feel like I was on a diet. I felt like I was on a lifestyle change. When I was on Weight Watchers the rules were too strict for me, because there were some days when I ate too much food in one category and I felt like that was the end of getting it right. And believe me, there are some days when I can eat ten pieces of fruit and not be done.

In all my dieting experiences before, I hadn't exercised, but Chris encouraged me to run, which was great. I followed the whole Peak 10, I took on the attitude that he was helping me so it was my obligation to help him. I was being real good about it. I was more religious with cardiovascular than I was with weights. If I didn't have time to do something I did the cardiovascular. I got myself up to two miles.

The only thing that was hard was exercising as much as I wanted to. I was fine during the summer, but indoor exercise bores me; but with the differences in my eating plan I've still kept the weight off. I only gained three pounds during the winter and I wasn't exercising.

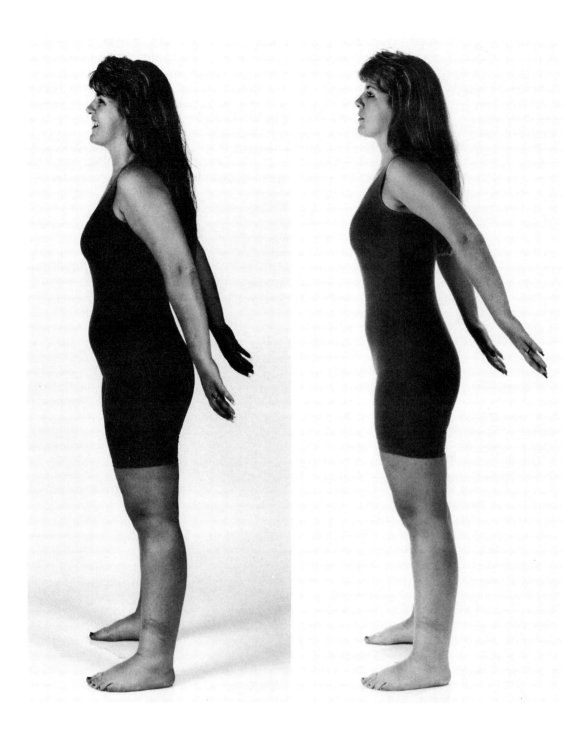

I noticed an incredible change in my energy level. I slept better and my head was clearer—and I didn't get one cold all winter. I'm getting married this spring so I'm getting into exercise again. My fiancé isn't concerned about my weight—whatever makes me happy is what matters. He was a big help in getting me running again and he helped me slow down. He comes with me if it's dark.

If I had a friend who wanted to lose some weight and get healthy, I would strongly suggest doing Peak 10. I've tried several things and this has been the best for me. If you follow everything the way you're supposed to, it will work.

Chris helped me learn why I could do this. There are certain things about weight and health that are factual—all you need is information. Peak 10 changed my lifestyle. I didn't start the program by saying that I would do this until I lost 15 pounds; instead, it was about learning things and taking advantage of what I was learning. It made me more energetic. It's a lot easier for me to get dressed and go out. I have things to wear that I feel good in. It's fabulous.

6

Tone Muscle, Burn More Fat

The strength and toning segment of the Peak 10 program is similar to a sculptor working with hammer and chisel to create an original sculpture. In this case you are the sculptor and your hammer and chisel are the exercises I have created especially for you. Working to build strength and definition has many rewards. Along with the obvious—looking great— you will also be improving your posture, maintaining bone density for the prevention of osteoporosis, and boosting your metabolism, causing your body to burn more fat, even at rest!

In the past there has been concern about the possible dangers of weight-bearing exercises, which has inhibited some people from maximizing their fitness goals. The most common concern among many women is the prospect of getting huge Schwarzenegger-type muscles. I assure you, it just won't happen. Even men have a tough time building muscles of that magnitude. It takes the right genes (being male) or a high level of male hormones as well as endless hours in the gym lifting heavy, heavy weights, so don't be concerned that you're going to bulk up if you're a woman.

Some other concerns are: How much weight should I use? How many times do I lift this weight? Are you sure I won't hurt myself? The list goes on and on. The bottom line is that you need to know exactly what to do. You need knowledge. With the knowledge that I'll provide and regular "perfect practice," you'll see very quick, impressive results. Best of all, the use of dumbbells, ankle weights, and a few trade secrets will change the shape of your body more quickly and more efficiently than any other means available. You gotta love that!

Here's some added evidence regarding training with weights. Wayne Westcott, National Strength Training Director for the YMCA, conducted a two-year study on five hundred clients, mostly women, and found that exercisers who combined weight training and aerobics lost two and a half times more fat than those who just did aerobics. Increasing your muscle mass increases your ability to burn fat.

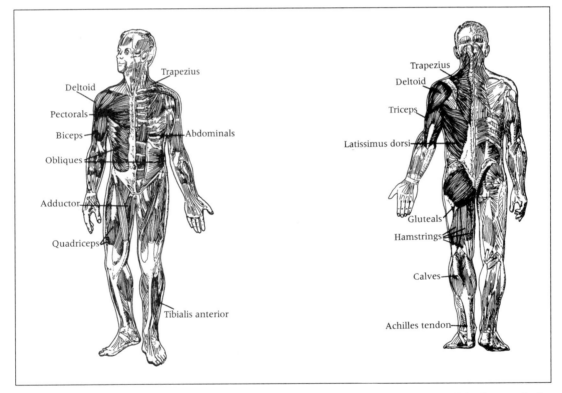

Front view of muscles of the human body.   *Back view of muscles of the human body.*

MOMENTARY MUSCULAR FAILURE, REPS AND SETS

Of course, strength training can only make a big difference in your body when you remember one of the key principles of Peak 10: knowledge. You need to master the proper techniques in order to maximize your efforts. I'll be more specific with individual exercises later on, but now I want to let you in on one of those trade secrets.

We don't gauge our workout by the time it takes. Instead, we aim to work our muscles to a point of failure—the precise moment when that five-pound dumbbell feels like a truck parked in your left hand. You need to understand that this is just a brief moment in time, and your discomfort will soon be over. Hence the term *momentary muscular failure*. This is a *good* thing. Practice will help you become familiar with the sensation of muscular failure. For most of us it is a shaky feeling in your muscle which may even burn slightly, until you don't have the strength left to do another repetition with perfect form. It is important to push yourself to that point in order to change. Your body will adapt to the increased stress placed on it by becoming stronger and more toned.

Along with momentary muscular failure, you'll need to add some new words to your fitness vocabulary. A *repetition,* or *"rep,"* is the act of performing one complete motion of a particular exercise. A complete repetition should take four to six seconds and you should breathe through it, exhaling as you exert pressure against a resistance. Never hold your breath. Equally important is keeping the weight steady: You don't want to "jerk" the weight up and then let it fall down. Strive for elegant motion—a slow, long motion.

A *set* is simply a group of reps of one exercise. For most of your routines, you will be performing high reps (between ten and twenty) with light weight, generally **one set** to failure. This approach will help to stimulate your muscles to be toned and tight.

MOVING THROUGH YOUR WORKOUT

Between every set of each exercise you will take time to rest and recover. Your *recovery period* will vary based upon your level of fitness and how you are feeling that particular day. By taking time (as long as you need, or as little as none when you are really "peaking") to rest between sets and catch your breath, you assure the maximum strength level for each contraction. You will maneuver through your workout, push your muscles to failure, rest the appropriate amount of time, and move on to the next exercise. You should note that if you shorten your recovery time, you will increase the intensity of the training. Turning up the intensity of the workout will help you to achieve your goals more quickly. Always remember to move at your pace and maintain a level of stress just above your comfort zone.

INTENSITY

There are two other ways to increase your training intensity. Adding more weight or doing more reps will force you to work harder. This portion of the program is based on your attaining momentary muscular failure. Setting the amount of resistance and the number of repetitions is more or less a test of trial and error. Let me remind you again, this is a ten-week program. Starting off slow, with little weights (three to five pounds for most women and eight to twenty pounds for most men) or no weight at all is exactly the way I want you to begin. Master the form and function of all the exercises before you start to boost the intensity. That's the way I do it with *all* my new clients.

FREQUENCY

The American College of Sports Medicine recommends that every one of us do some form of strength training twice a week in order to maintain functional strength. But you and I are aiming higher than just functional strength. I want you to be in the best shape of your life. To that end I have designed, in conjunction with your fat-burning and cardiovascular workouts, a series of three strength and toning workouts per week. The workouts are spaced apart with at least thirty-six hours between each one. This downtime assures ample recovery for optimum results.

CHOOSING YOUR WEAPONS (WEIGHTS, THAT IS)

I recommend that you start your program with weights that are light enough to practice the form of each exercise that requires added weight. Three to five pounds is perfect even if you've weight-trained before. I want you to polish your form before you add more weight. Knowing the proper form of the exercise is what counts in the beginning. Take the time to learn and practice. When you can complete all the exercises easily (that is, if you can finish the number of reps and go on to do more), move on to heavier weights.

When using dumbbells and other free weights, you're forced to involve other surrounding muscles to aid and support as well as stabilize the working area. Free weights also allow your body to move in a natural range of motion. Your muscles will benefit from these types of weights and exercises, because you're forced to balance the weights. This is not the case when working with weight machines.

That's not to say that weight machines don't have their place. If you have the luxury of using some exercise machines (with guidance) during your Peak 10 program, by all means take advantage of it.

"SLOW AND CONTROLLED"

Imagine that from a standstill you're going to jump up in the air. You squat down a little, push off, and you're up. Even though your feet leave the ground, you still keep moving up because of the momentum you've created. You've stopped using your own energy, and your muscles are no longer contracting, but you still keep rising. Relying on momentum is *not* the best way to create stronger, sleeker muscles. That's why we do our exercises in a *slow and controlled* manner. It's a great little mantra to use while you're lifting weights or using machines because it describes exactly the way you should move the working muscles. Exercising in a slow and controlled manner will greatly reduce your risk of injury, which is particularly important if you have a preexisting condition. Control is also important to help you to isolate particular muscles or groups of muscles.

IT'S ABOUT YOU

You're moving through your workouts at your own pace. This is what makes the program customized and this is what makes it personal. You want momentary muscular failure without compromising your form. The second you feel you're struggling and using perhaps your lower back or some other part of your body, that's an indication that you've reached your goal. As long as you're controlling the weights, and not having the weights control you, you're okay.

I've provided a daily, easy-to-use training log in chapters 8 through 10. Keep track of your weights and the number of reps. Use these numbers to establish your progress. Track your progress and push to outperform your last attempt at a particular exercise—that's what it's all about. Keep getting better!

If you work out at a gym or if you use my Peak 10 videos, remember, you're competing against no one but yourself. Move at your own pace. When the weights you're using start feeling lighter, don't speed up! A trick I use with my clients and in my own workouts is to *slow down* the speed of the reps. Slowing down the repetitions will make you work a little harder, especially at the tail end of the set.

As Always, Listen to Your Body

Since the key to your weight-training session is to push to momentary muscular failure within ten to twenty reps with the correct weight for each exercise, this is another opportunity for you to really listen to your body. You want to feel it! I'm not talking about pain, I'm talking about the isolation and total contraction of the muscle or muscle groups being worked. When you lift or pull on a weight, are you feeling the strain in your forearm when you are trying to work your biceps? Are you tensing your shoulders when you're doing your lunges? My point is that I want you to become fully aware of your entire body. Pay close attention to your posture, the position of your hips, knees, and feet. Go through a checklist with yourself. This will reinforce everything you are learning. It only works if you understand what you're doing.

Spot Reducing vs. Spot Shaping

No doubt you already have in mind the body parts you're looking forward to changing. Perhaps you want thinner thighs or a higher rear end. In fact, it is possible to sculpt your body with the proper use of weights and other muscle-toning exercises. While aerobics can give you a stronger heart and help boost the number of calories you burn, only strength training can truly redefine your body.

While spot *shaping* is a great way to focus on the body parts that you want to improve, it is imperative that you understand that *you cannot spot-reduce.* In order to reduce, you need to lower your entire body-fat percentage—that means all over your body. No number of sit-ups will burn the fat that you have around your waist. Aerobic exercise and proper diet are the *only* way to lose the fat.

Let me let you in on another little trade secret. *You cannot turn fat to muscle,* or vice versa for that matter. Muscle is muscle, and fat is fat. When muscle is not stimulated by resistance, it simply withers away. The bummer about this is that because muscle is what drives our metabolism, you are burning fewer calories when you lose muscle. Lose muscle, lower metabolism, gain fat. The bonus about muscle is that when it is stimulated, even if dormant for years, it can be regenerated by weight training. Gain muscle, raise metabolism, lose fat. Get it?

YOU'RE GOING TO THE TOP

Since you'll be on Peak 10 for ten weeks, your body will get stronger and more fit each and every day. To keep your body from adapting to the workouts, I've divided the ten weeks into three sections. During each section you'll do a stretching and strength-training routine three days per week. Remember to go slowly. Shoot for fifteen to twenty reps of each exercise, working to momentary muscular failure.

I designed Peak 10 as if you were setting out to climb a mountain. Like climbing a mountain, you will be starting at the bottom, or as I call it, Base Camp. You'll be at Base Camp for the first three weeks, learning and developing the skills it will take to make the climb to the top. At week four, your body will become more accustomed to the routines of the program and you will continue your climb upward to the "Midway Ascent." Midway Ascent is the core of the Peak 10 program and makes up weeks four through seven. As you near the top of your climb and ascend to the peak, you will be challenged by the "Peak Circuit." For the last three weeks of the program you will be tested on your experiences and what you have learned and practiced.

THE BASIC EXERCISES EXPLAINED

Forget the image you have in your mind of overdeveloped weight lifters with their tense faces and popping veins. The first step to picking up a weight is to relax. The first step to doing a strength-building exercise *without* weights is also to relax. Take a deep breath and give yourself time. Stand naturally. If you suspect that your posture needs help, try to do the exercises in front of a mirror or have a friend help you stay in position. All of these exercises, especially the ones for your back and stomach, will help improve your posture, but it's a good idea to learn what good form is as soon as possible. Here are some hints:

- When standing, stand with your feet about hip distance apart. Your position should feel natural and not stressed. Relax and bend your knees slightly. Keep your abdominals tight and face forward. This is the neutral position.
- When doing any exercise, even if you're bent over a chair, try to keep your back straight. Bending your knees or placing your feet in an up position will help keep your back well supported by the surrounding muscles.
- Try putting your shoulders back and down. Most of us bend forward with our chest and shoulders. I hated hearing it too, but "sit up straight."
- Keep your wrists straight—not bent up or down or side to side—when holding a weight. If they're not straight, it could cause undue stress and fatigue in the muscles of the forearm and might keep you from working the muscle that you're trying to work.
- Get a grip. Using gloves designed for weight training will prevent calluses as well as help to reduce hand and forearm fatigue.

STRETCH . . . BEFORE YOU STRESS

To avoid injury, it is important to warm up your muscles. We warm up before aerobic activity by going slow for the first five or fifteen minutes. When it comes to strength training, you will be warming up through a series of stretches. Here's what they should look like:

Neck Stretch (back)

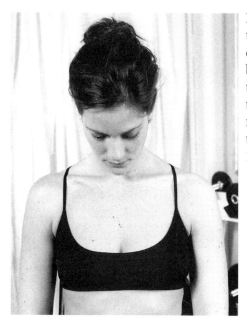

Begin by standing in a neutral position. Be sure to keep your shoulders relaxed and knees slightly bent. Slowly bow your head down toward your chest. You needn't touch your chin to your chest if it is not comfortable, but if you can, that's fine too. Hold that for 15 to 30 seconds.

Neck Stretch (side)

Remain in the neutral standing position. Look right while keeping your shoulders straight. Don't turn your head past a point that feels comfortable enough to hold for 15 to 30 seconds. Turn your head left and hold for the same amount of time. Repeat all three neck stretches at least two times.

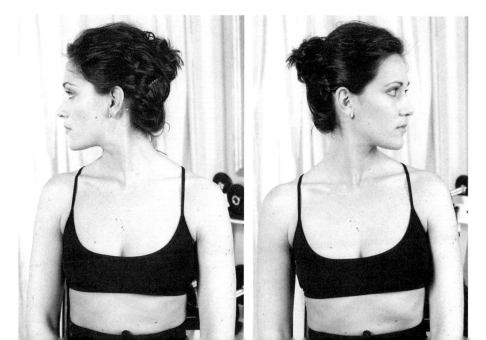

Chest/Biceps

Stand in a neutral position near a stationary pole or door. Grasp the pole or door with your hand and turn your body in the opposite direction until you feel a stretch in your chest and arm. Repeat the same stretch with the other arm. Hold 15 to 30 seconds and repeat.

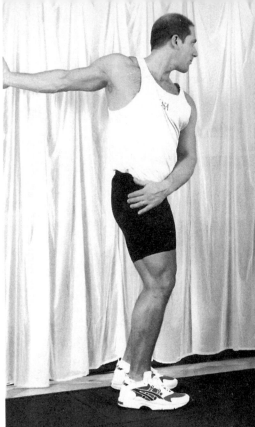

Shoulder/Upper Back

Stand in a neutral position. Cross one arm in front of your chest. Grasp that arm at the elbow with your opposite hand. Pull the arm further across your chest, being careful to keep your shoulders down. Repeat with the other arm. Hold 15 to 30 seconds on each side and repeat.

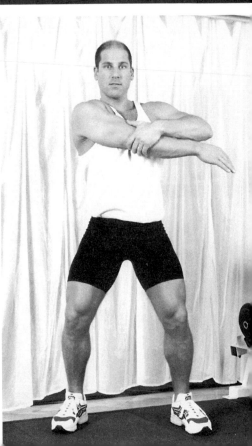

Modified Hurdler Stretch

Lower yourself gently to the floor. Sit with one leg straight in front of you, and the other bent at the knee against the floor. Lean forward without bouncing until you feel a good stretch through the back of your leg. If you can't reach your toes, you can use a towel to pull your toe toward you gently. Reverse legs and repeat. Hold 15 to 30 seconds on each leg and repeat.

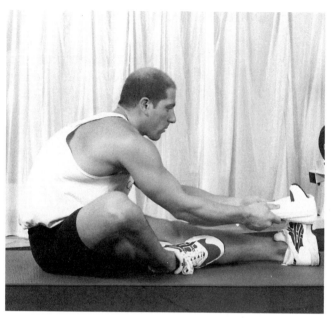

Flat Back Hamstring

Begin by lying on your back flat on the floor. Slowly raise one leg with knee slightly bent until you can grasp it behind the thigh. Flex your toes as you gently pull your leg toward your head. When you can't pull any closer without discomfort, hold it there for 15 to 30 seconds. Now stretch the other leg and repeat.

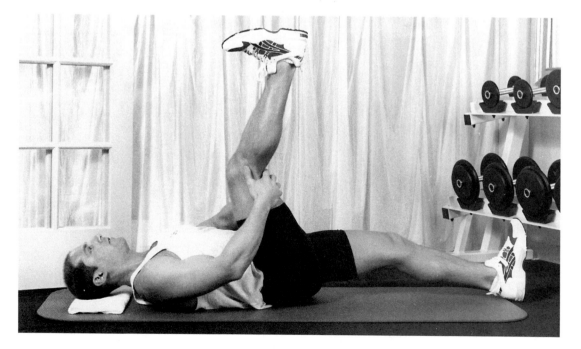

Double Knee to Chest

Lying flat on your back on the floor, curl your knees up to your chest. Hold your legs in place behind your knees for a good 15-to-30-second stretch and repeat.

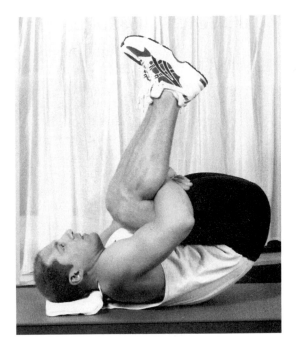

Side Quad Stretch

From the position flat on your back on the floor, roll to one side and hold. For stabilization, bend the knee that is touching the floor as you grab the foot of the opposite leg. Pull toward your butt and hold for 15 to 30 seconds. Roll to the other side and repeat. Then go back and stretch each side once more.

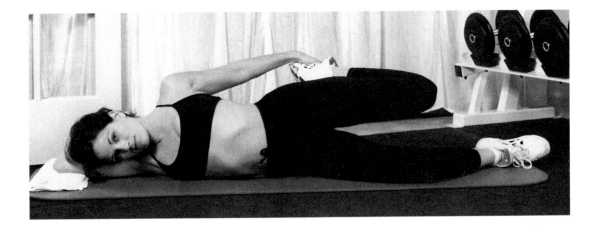

Child Stretch

This is a great one for your back. From a prone position, pull your knees underneath your body as you stretch your arms overhead and rest your arms and your head on the floor. Exaggerate the stretch by pulling forward with your hands. Hold this for 15 to 30 seconds.

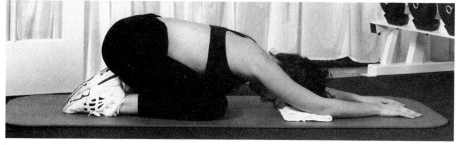

Calf Stretch

From a standing position, grab something stable to help balance you. With one foot flat on the floor, extend the opposite leg one step in front of you and rest on your heel. Be sure to keep both knees slightly bent throughout. Push down against the floor with your outstretched leg. Hold for 15 to 30 seconds and repeat with the opposite leg. Then repeat with each leg again.

Now let's see exactly how the exercises should be done.

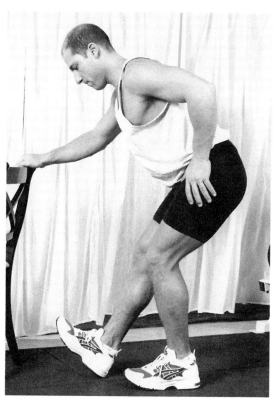

EXERCISES FOR WEEKS ONE THROUGH THREE

BASE CAMP

LEG AND BUTT EXERCISES

Leg Extension

This exercise works the front of the thigh.

Stand beside a chair, holding the top rail with your hand. Don't clench your fingers. Relax. Keep your feet hip width apart. Support yourself with your left leg (keep left knee slightly bent) while raising your right knee, holding foot and calf at a 90-degree angle at the knee. This is the starting position. From this position, move to straighten your right leg with your toe pointed, attempting to achieve full extension. Don't be surprised if you can't extend fully; this is perfectly normal. Keep your hips steady, only move your leg. Remember: slow and controlled. Your leg should go only as high as is comfortable. Hold the top position and lower your leg to the starting position and do 15 to 20 reps, then change to the other leg. As you advance, try using an ankle weight to add resistance.

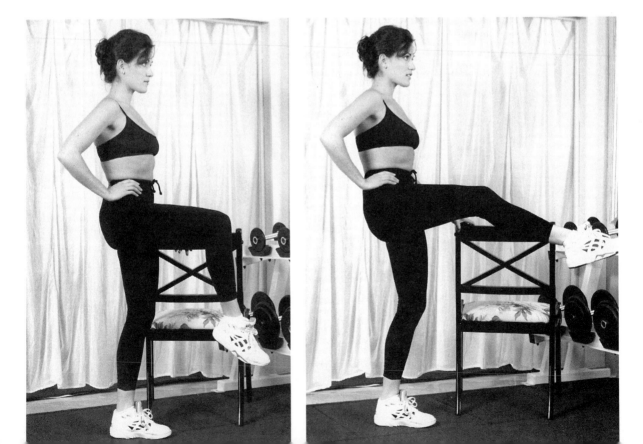

Leg Curl

This exercise works your hamstrings (the back of your thigh).

Stand behind a chair, holding the top with both hands. Keep your feet hip width apart. Bend over the chair slightly, without leaning on it too heavily. Don't clench your fingers. Stay relaxed. Extend one leg back and pull your heel up toward your rear end. Remember: slow and controlled. It's easy to "swing" your leg up, but that won't work the muscle as much. Repeat this 15 to 20 times, then change to the other leg.

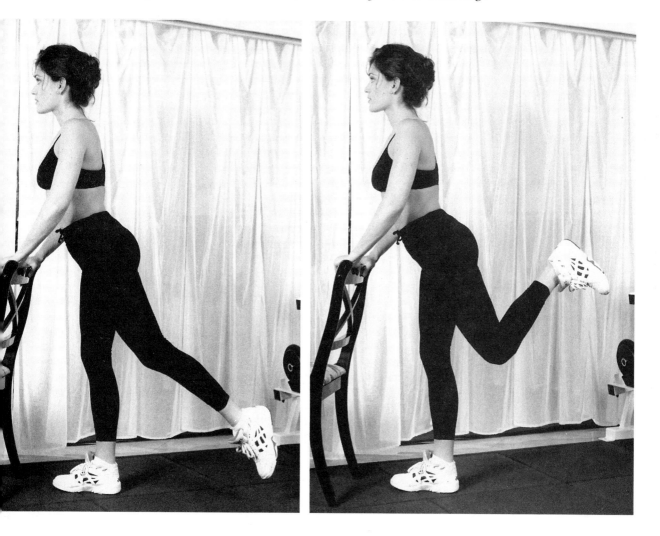

Plié

This exercise works the front of your upper leg as well as your butt and inner thigh.

This is a traditional exercise from ballet. You can hold onto a chair or do it without support. Either way, start with your feet slightly more than hip width apart—far enough so that when you bend your knees and lower your butt, your knees don't extend past your toes. Stand with your butt tucked under (that is, be sure your hips aren't swaying back). Your feet should be turned out (toes pointed away from your body). With abs tight and back straight, lower your buttocks, until your knees are bent to a 90-degree angle, so that your thighs are parallel to the floor.

Now slowly straighten your knees, but it should be as if your head is leading the way, moving up toward a standing position. As you rise, you should feel the muscles in your inner thighs and your buttocks tighten. Lower back down. Now you should feel the muscles in the tops of your legs. Repeat this 15 to 20 times.

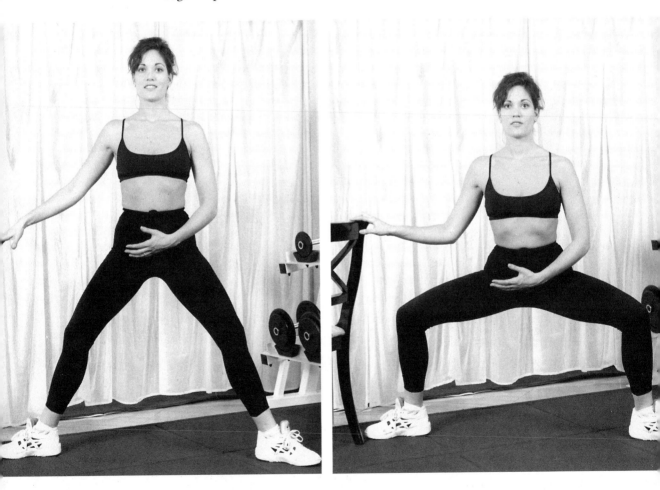

CHEST, ARM, AND BACK EXERCISES

Chest Press

This strengthens the muscles in your chest, shoulders, and triceps.

You'll need hand weights for this exercise.

   Lie on your back with a pillow beneath your back, shoulders, and head. Your legs should be bent, feet flat on the floor so that your lower back is firm against the floor. Hold a weight in each hand. Start with your elbows out to the sides with hands positioned over elbows. Raise the weights up and center without locking your elbows or rotating your shoulders. You should feel the muscles in your chest and arms bearing the weight. Lower the weights to the starting position and repeat. Do 15 to 20 repetitions. Rest the weights on your stomach between sets.

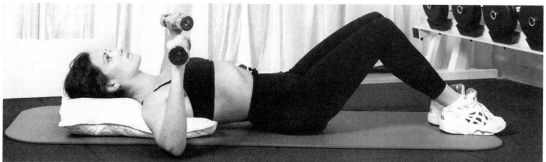

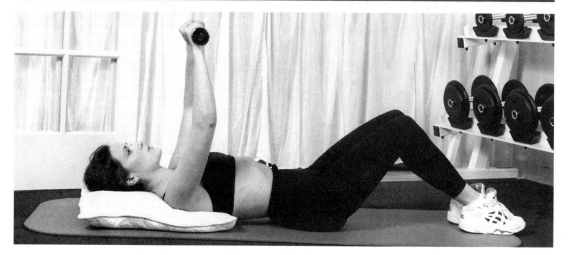

Chest Fly

This exercise works the chest (pectorals).

You'll need hand weights for this exercise.

Lie on your back with a pillow beneath your back, shoulders, and head, with arms extended over your chest, with a slightly exaggerated bend in the elbow and palms facing each other. Slowly lower the weights, maintaining the slightly bent elbow, until your elbows are even with your shoulders. The movement should resemble hugging a beach ball. Hold bottom position briefly and return to top center position. Repeat this 15 to 20 times. Rest the weights on your stomach between sets.

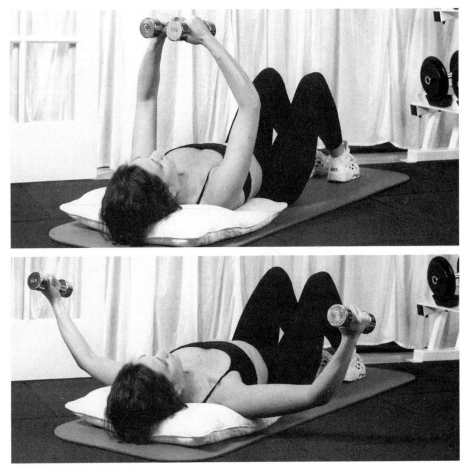

Bent-Over Row

This exercise is great for the muscles of the back (the latissimus dorsi).

You'll need hand weights for this exercise.

   With a weight in one hand and arm fully extended, position the same-side leg back for balance. Hold your upper body steady, with your opposite hand resting on a chair. Keep your neck aligned with your spine. Keep knees bent, toes forward, and elbows bent slightly. Make certain to keep your abs tight and hips low for lower back support. Raise weight toward hip by bending and raising your elbow. Pause, hold the up position, then lower weight down to starting position. Repeat and switch sides. Do 15 to 20 reps on each side.

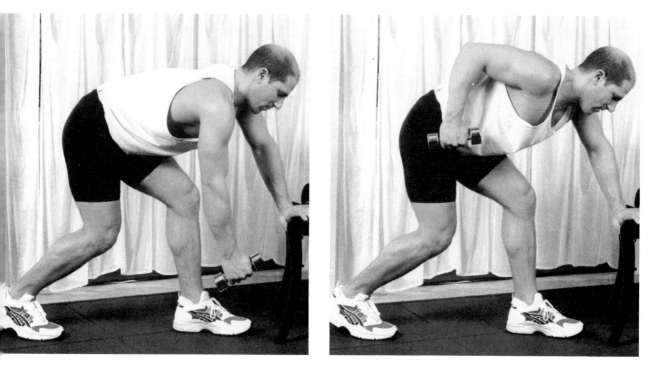

Upright Row

This works the muscles of the upper back and shoulders (trapezius and deltoids).

You'll need hand weights for this exercise.

Stand with a weight in each hand, your palms facing your body just in front of your thighs. Like most of the upright exercises, keep your knees slightly bent and your abdominals tight. With eyes forward, start motion by raising your elbows up and out. Don't try to overlift by bending your wrists. Your hands are there to hold the weight and go along for the ride. Inhale as you lift. Keep your shoulders relaxed. Exhale as you lower your arms and repeat. Do this 15 to 20 times.

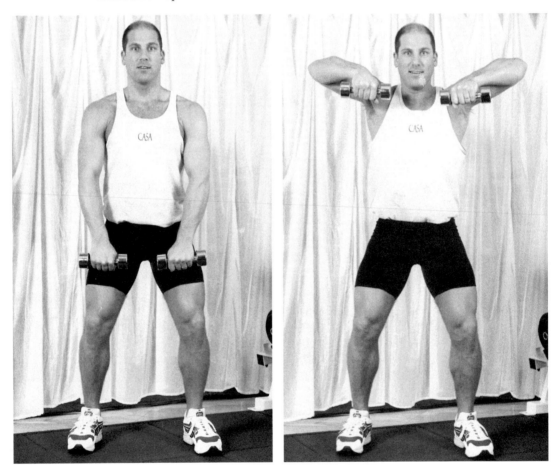

Lateral Raise

You'll need hand weights for this exercise.

Stand up, arms at your sides, a weight in each hand. Be sure your neck is relaxed. Look straight ahead. With elbows slightly bent through a full range of motion, raise your arms out to your sides, making sure your shoulders don't rise up toward your ears. Only raise your arms to just below shoulder level. Slow and controlled, as always. Lower them back down. Try for 15 to 20 repetitions.

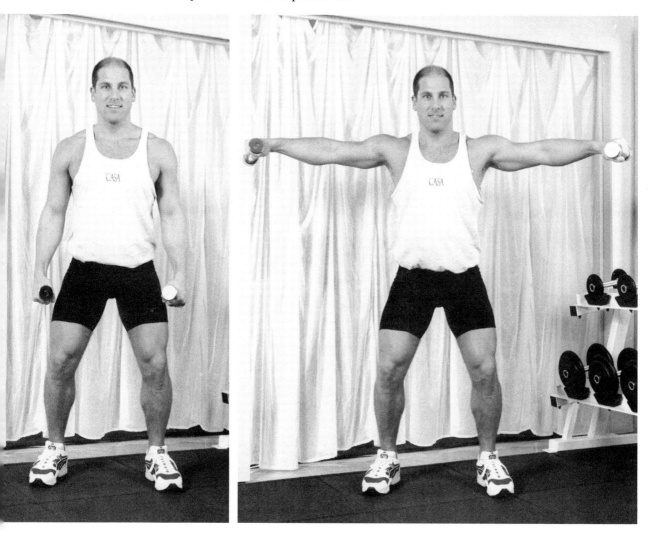

Biceps Curl

Your biceps are the muscles in the front of your upper arm. Combining this exercise with the Triceps Extension will create flab-free arms.

You'll need hand weights for this exercise.

Stand in the neutral position holding hand weights. Keep your elbows close to your sides, your palms facing up. Don't arch your back, keep abs tight. Raise your hands up toward your shoulders, squeeze tight (flex, make the connection), then lower them back down. Do this 15 to 20 times.

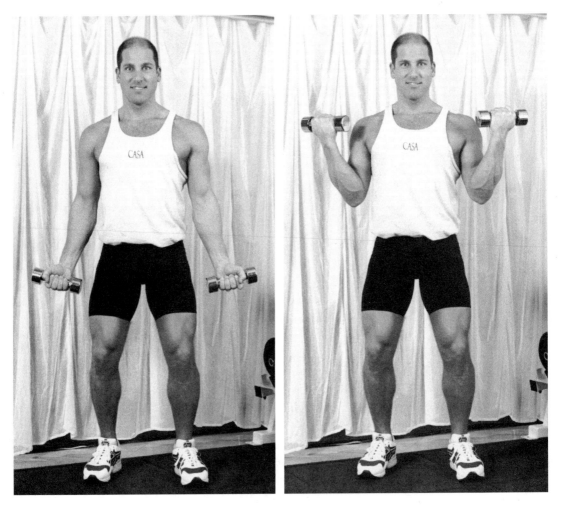

Triceps Extension

Your triceps are the muscles in the back of your upper arm. With a reduction in body fat and this exercise, you will have totally toned arms.

You'll need a hand weight for this exercise.

Stand in the neutral position and cup the end of a dumbbell with both hands. Raise your arms over your head, lowering your hands behind your head. This is the starting point of the exercise. Now raise your hands, straightening your arms. Keep your shoulders down, knees bent and abs tight. At the end of the exercise your arms will be straight above your head. Lower the weight back down. Be careful not to hit your head. Do this 15 to 20 times.

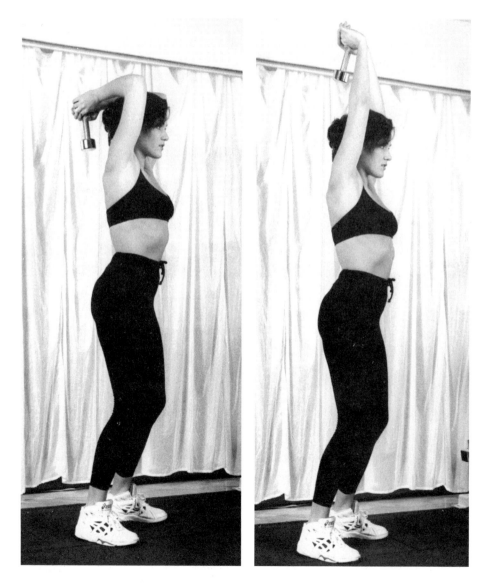

Abdominal Crunch

This exercise focuses on the abdominals. Your abdominals are the anchors of the body. They help to support and protect the lower back.

Lie on your back with your feet flat on the floor, knees bent. Be sure to keep your lower back flat on the floor. Place your hands on your thighs. Keep your eyes focused just past your knees and lift your upper body in that direction. You want to move about 10 inches total. Don't try to sit up all the way, and, on the way down, don't drop your body to the floor; maintain constant tension on the abdominal muscles. Remember: slow and controlled. Aim for at least 20 repetitions, work to failure: This is where you set the limit. Should your neck become fatigued, try supporting your head with your fingertips. This ensures that you won't be lifting your head with your hands. (If your neck is fatiguing on a regular basis, it needs to be strengthened. Try lifting your head, eyes to the ceiling, about an inch from the floor and hold it for 5 to 10 seconds. Do this for 3 sets, 3 times a week.)

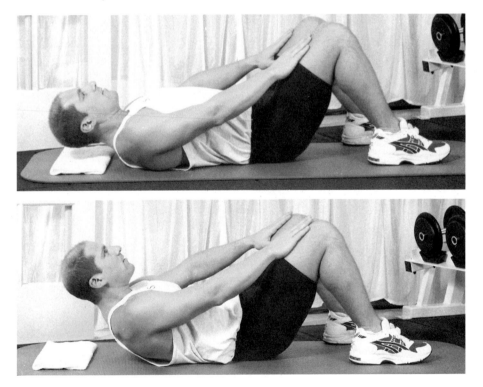

Prone Hyperextension #1

This is a great exercise to strengthen the lower back. It's an adaptation of a yoga move.

Lie on your stomach with your forehead on the floor. Your arms should be at your sides with palms facing up. Inhale slowly and on the exhale raise shoulders, head, and chest off the floor about 6 inches. Keep your eyes to the floor and hold the top for 1 second and then lower yourself slowly back to the floor. Do this 5 to 10 times, eventually working your way up to 20. If you have lower back limitations, check with your doctor before doing this.

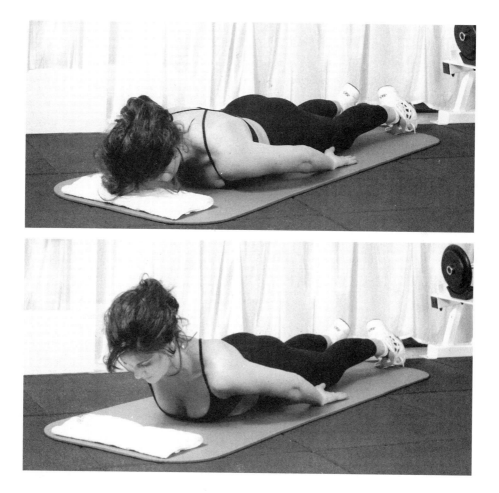

EXERCISES (ADDED) FOR WEEKS FOUR THROUGH SEVEN

MIDWAY ASCENT

The principles here are the same as in the introductory set. You should still do 15 to 20 repetitions in each set. As always, work to momentary muscular failure in a slow and controlled fashion. Don't forget to rest 30 to 60 seconds between exercises.

NEW EXERCISES

Lunge

Lunges work your thighs and butt. They require a lot of balance, though, so if you feel like you're wobbling too much, try doing the lunges while holding onto a chair.

Position yourself with one foot forward, keeping your back straight. Lower your back knee toward the floor without letting it touch. Your opposite thigh should be parallel to the floor. Make sure your knee doesn't go past your toe. Raise your body back to the standing position without locking your knees. Do one leg at a time, completing 15 to 20 repetitions on each side. Hand weights can be held for added resistance as you progress.

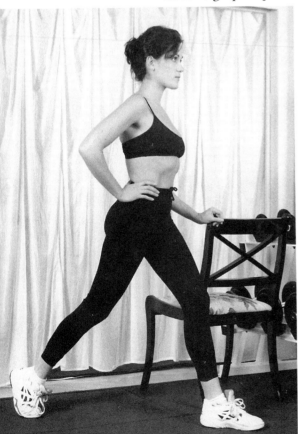

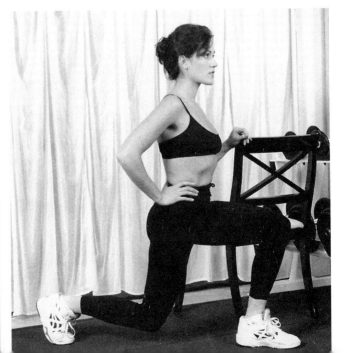

Plié Slide

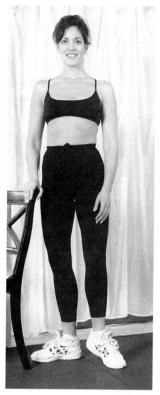

This exercise works the thighs and butt just like a regular plié, but the slide works your inner thigh to a greater degree.

This is a more advanced move than our basic plié. You'll need a chair for balance. Start with feet close together and toes turned out. With knees slightly bent, step to the side with one leg, maintaining the toe-out position. Gently, and with complete control, step one foot out to a position where your feet are 2 to 3 feet apart (the longer your legs, the greater the distance). Touch down as if you're doing a regular plié, lowering your buttocks toward the floor. Instead of raising your body straight up, slide or drag the extended toe back to the starting position. Keep your torso straight while you're moving so that in the final pose you're standing up straight, legs together. Do 15 to 20 repetitions, then switch to the other leg.

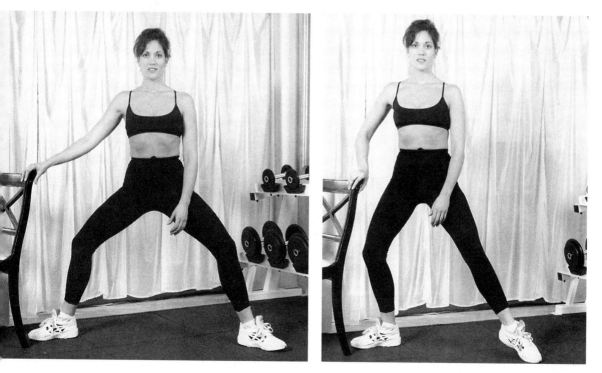

Reverse Lunge

Like the forward lunge, this exercise works your legs and butt, just a little variety to spice things up. Once again, you need a lot of balance, so don't hesitate to hold onto a chair.

Stand with your feet hip width apart and raise one knee to hip level. Swing that same leg back and behind you, lowering your knee toward—but not to—the floor. Don't let your other knee extend past your toe. Bring your leg back up to the starting position. Be sure not to arch your back as you raise your leg. Repeat each leg 15 to 20 times.

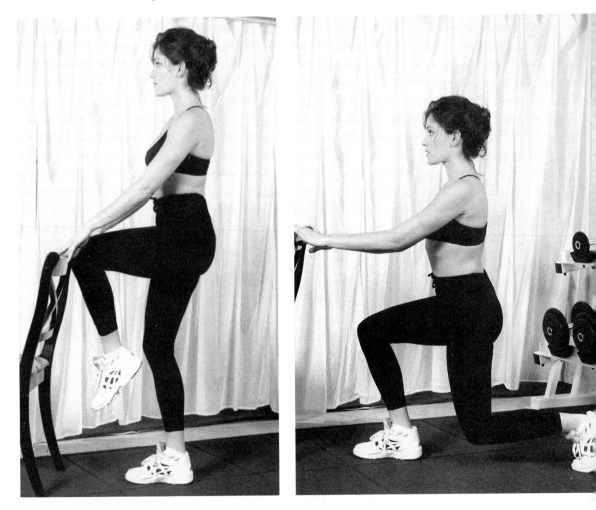

Outer Thigh

As the name states, this exercise focuses on your outer thigh.

From the neutral position and balanced behind a chair, slightly bend one knee so that you are on your toes. Raise that leg up to the side as high as it will go without turning your hips. Hold the top position and lower without resting your toes on the floor. The slower you do this motion without swinging it, the more effective it is. Repeat 15 to 20 times, then switch sides and work the other leg.

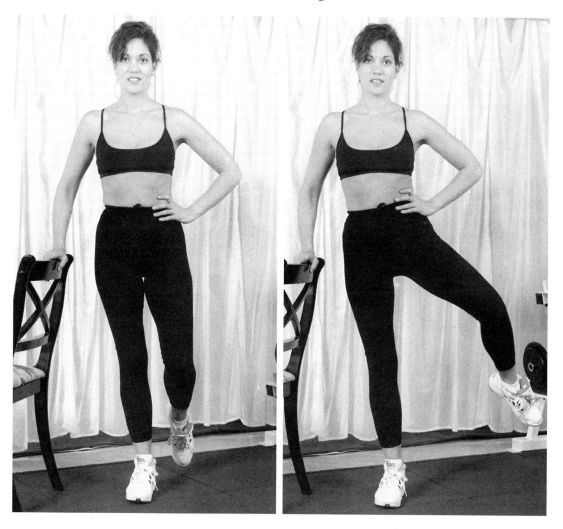

Overhead Press

This is another exercise for your shoulders. It also incorporates your triceps.

You'll need hand weights for this exercise.

This exercise is extra challenging, so start with little or no weight. Stand with your feet hip width apart, body straight. Hold a weight in each hand, weights over elbows, elbows slightly below shoulder level (your arms are bent). Slowly raise the weights over your head, straightening your arms (but don't lock your elbows). Be sure to keep your shoulders in place. Lower your hands slowly to the starting position. Do this about 15 to 20 times.

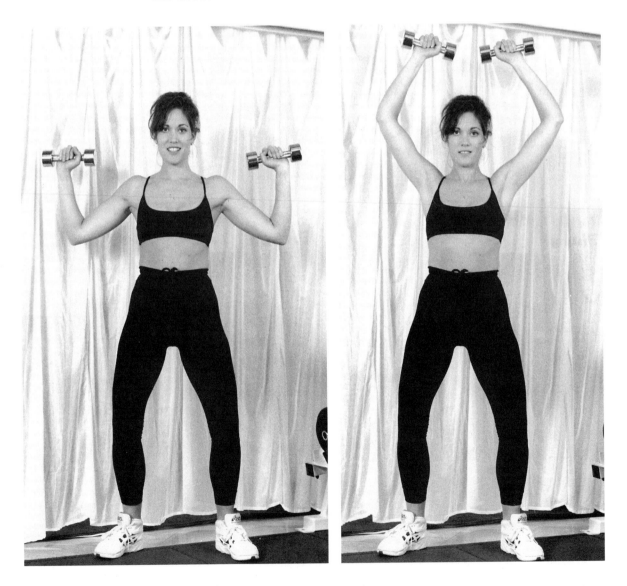

Side Crunch

This exercise works the abdominal muscles that run along the sides of your torso. They're called the obliques.

Lie on your back with your fingertips placed on your head behind your ears. Your knees should be bent and resting on one side. Keep your body open, chest up, as you raise your shoulders toward your hip. This is a small, concentrated movement upward. Maintain neck alignment by keeping your eyes toward the ceiling. Repeat this 15 to 20 times on each side.

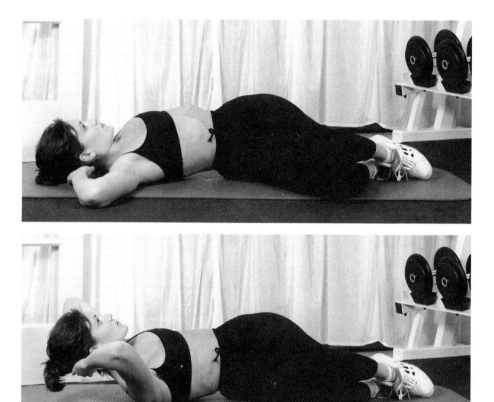

Reverse Crunch

This is another abdominal exercise, with focus on the lower portion of your abdominal muscle.

Lie on your back, legs up in the air, with knees slightly bent. Put your arms to the sides with palms down. Raise your rear end and hips off the floor very slightly (about 2 inches), lifting your feet toward the ceiling. Don't swing your legs. The slower you do this, the harder the muscles will work. You'll really feel it after a few reps—aim for 15 to 20.

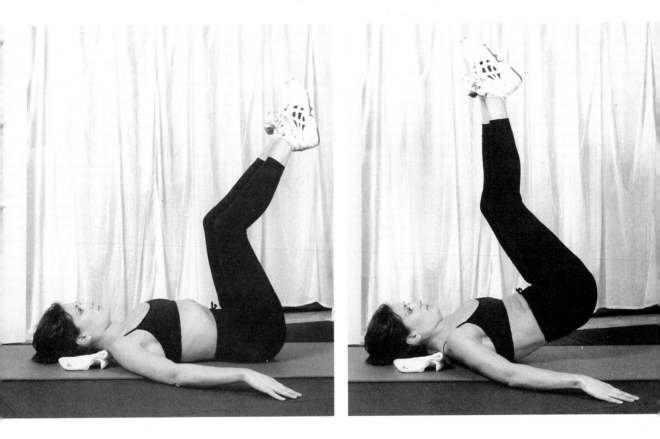

Prone Hyperextension #2

This is an advanced version of the Prone Hyperextension #1. It strengthens the lower back as well.

Lie on your stomach, this time with your forehead resting on the tops of your hands. The weight of your arms will increase the resistance of the exercise. Inhale slowly and on the exhale raise your arms, shoulders, head, and chest off the floor about 6 inches. Keep your eyes to the floor and hold the top for 1 second and then lower yourself slowly back to the floor. Do 5 to 10 reps, eventually working your way to 20. If you have lower back problems, check with your doctor before doing this exercise.

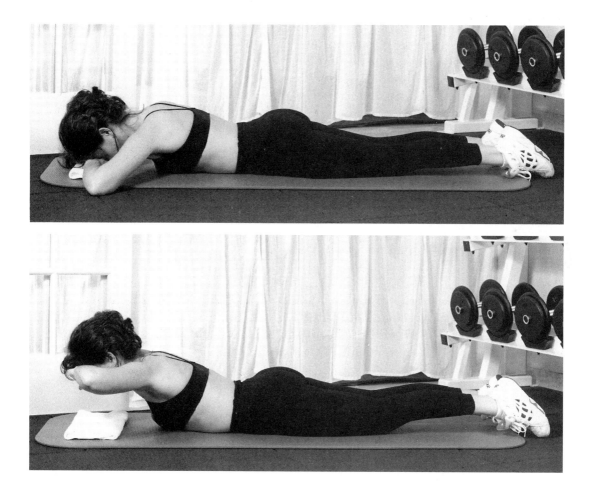

EXERCISES FOR WEEKS EIGHT THROUGH TEN

PEAK CIRCUIT

By now you're becoming more fit, and with all the practice you've had, you could probably do these exercises in your sleep. You can also do this workout with much shorter rests between sets, so be sure all of your weights are close at hand. I want you to shoot for 20 to 30 reps of each exercise, slow and controlled. Rest from 15 to 30 seconds between sets.

LUNGE (see description)
CHEST PRESS (see description)
LEG EXTENSION (see description)
BENT-OVER ROW (see description)
LEG CURL (see description)
UPRIGHT ROW (see description)
PLIÉ SLIDE (see description)
OVERHEAD PRESS (see description)
REVERSE LUNGE (see description)
BICEPS CURL (see description)
OUTER THIGH (see description)
TRICEPS DIP (see description)
ABDOMINAL CRUNCH (see description)
SIDE CRUNCH (see description)
REVERSE CRUNCH (see description)
PRONE HYPEREXTENSION #2 (see description)

HOT SPOTS

These are exercise routines that focus on a particular body part. If you have a particular body part that needs some extra help, here's the ammo. Do these as extra credit in addition to your daily assignment or where indicated on your training schedule.

BUTT

LUNGE (see description)
LEG CURL (see description)
PLIÉ (see description)
REVERSE LUNGE (see description)

Heel-Ups

This exercise really works the gluteals—the muscles in your butt.

Stand behind a chair facing its back, holding the top loosely with your hands. Lean forward a little but don't rest on the chair. Bend one leg behind you, flexing your foot. Move your leg back and slightly up from your body, heel toward the ceiling. If you put your hand on your rear end, you can feel the muscle moving. Lower your knee back in maintaining the angle of the knee of the leg you are working throughout this exercise. Repeat this about 15 to 20 times, slowly, then switch to the other leg.

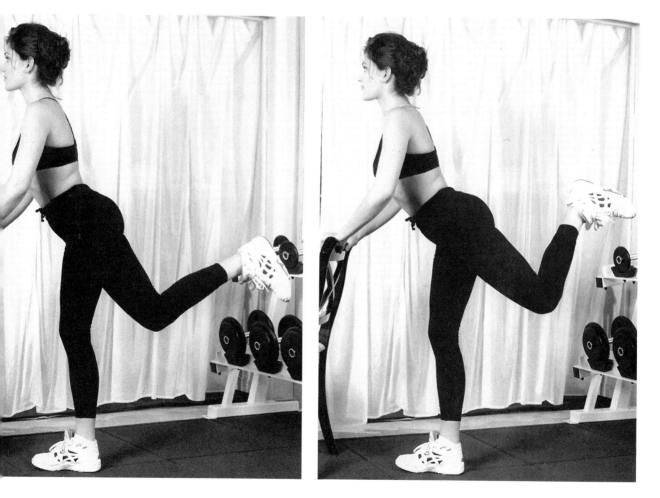

ARMS

BICEPS CURL (see description)
TRICEPS EXTENSION (see description)

Triceps Dip

This is a more advanced exercise that works the backs of the arms.

Stand in front of a chair, grasping the seat behind you with your palms. Your feet should be far enough from the chair to allow your butt to be lowered toward the floor. You can vary the intensity by moving your feet further away from the chair: The further away your feet are, the more difficult the exercise will be. Lower yourself to the floor, bending your elbows, keeping your back straight while supporting your weight with your arms. Lower yourself to the point where your shoulders are level with your elbows. There's no need to go further down than that. Return to top position and repeat 15 to 20 times. This is a pretty tough exercise. Do the best that you can and monitor your progress.

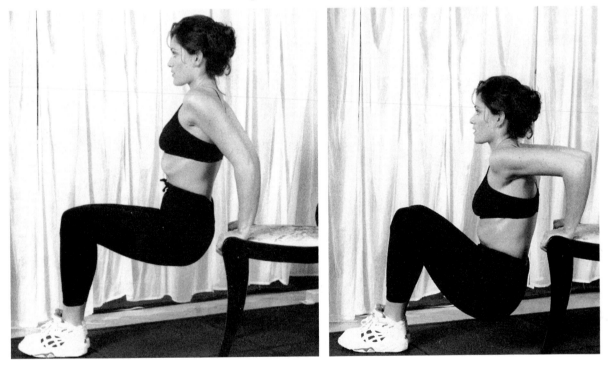

ABDOMINALS

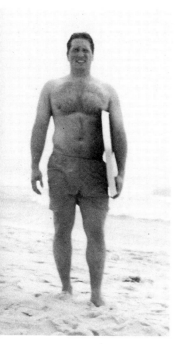

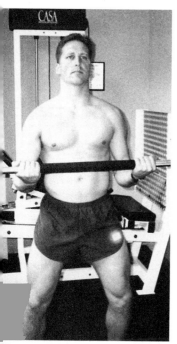

ABDOMINAL CRUNCH (see description)
SIDE CRUNCH (see description)
REVERSE CRUNCH (see description)
PRONE HYPEREXTENSION #2 (see description)

THOMAS'S STORY

Thomas
Age: 29
Height: 5'9"

	Start	Finish
Weight	212 lbs.	178 lbs.
% Fat	18%	9.2%

This is Thomas. If he looks familiar, that's probably because he is my little brother. But he looked more like my "big" brother last year. Like many people, Tom was much more active in school, and then became sedentary when he started working. There were too many other things in his life that were taking priority over his physical well-being. And believe me, I hounded him about it.

When I started my gym, I asked Thomas to come work for me. And he did. Thomas doesn't look the way he does in his "after" picture because he works out all day—I don't give him the time. But I will tell you that he trains with weights three times a week, does some cardio work three to five times a week, and pays much more attention to his eating habits. He eats lots of fresh fruit, vegetables, and lean protein. And he drinks plenty of water.

I'm not saying that you have to become a trainer to get into shape. But Thomas is a good example of someone who made changes in his body by becoming more active. If you know what changes to make, that's half the battle. Make a plan and stick to it and you, too, can look back at old photos and feel proud of how you look now.

7

Putting Your Plan Together

We've learned a lot in the last six chapters, and it's time to start pulling it together and turning it into your *personal* Peak 10 program. The first step is to look over what you've done with your Dietary Recall.

EVALUATING YOUR DIETARY RECALL

By now you might have had time to fill in some, or all, of the seven days. Don't try to fill it out all in one day because you won't be able to remember what you ate. Most people can't even remember what they've eaten over the course of the *day,* much less a whole week. I've had several clients hand in their Dietary Recall after a week, and I can see from the writing that they did it all in one day, or they left huge gaps in it. When this happens, I give them a new book and make them do it again. The people who don't fill out the Dietary Recall correctly have much less of a chance of succeeding at Peak 10.

Counting calories and fat grams is tedious, I know. But luckily it is only half of the Peak 10 dietary equation. The other part is to teach you to learn more about you and your eating habits. As you can see by the Dietary Recall, I'm interested in what you eat, when you eat, how much you eat, and how you feel when you eat. This isn't about deprivation or feeling bad about yourself. It's about helping yourself. I want you to look at the quality of your meals as a whole.

When you have completed your Dietary Recall, take a look at the way you ate over the past week and see what you think. I bet that I don't need to say anything: You probably already know what you're doing to keep from being lean and fit. (If you feel you need a refresher course on healthful eating, go back and read chapters 3 and 4 again. There's a lot of complicated information in there that you might want to review before going over your Dietary Recall.)

The first thing that we're going to look at is the *content of your food.* I want you to examine the types of foods that you're eating. Are they high in fat? If you don't know, get a calorie counter and look them up. If they are, think of some other low-fat choices that you could have made instead. Choose skim or nonfat milk rather than whole milk, and that applies to all dairy products. Snack on pickles rather than olives, pretzels rather than potato chips, make grilled fish or chicken rather than pork or beef.

Did you eat a lot of sweets? Don't forget, sugar can make you fat too. Try to change your habits slowly and distinctly to improve what you're putting into your mouth. Other things to look for: Are you eating your vegetables and fruit? Is your body getting enough fiber? You know how great fiber can be for you, and how rotten you'll feel if you don't eat enough. Take a spin through your kitchen and get an idea of what it is that you have to choose from. If your selection is lousy, take the grocery list that I made for you and go shopping.

Did you drink lots of water? Don't forget to "keep it clear."

The next thing that I want you to look at in your Dietary Recall is your *frequency of meals.* You can easily spot patterns of skipping breakfast, for example. Try to figure out why you're doing this. Are you too rushed? Maybe you need to get up a little earlier, or stop and get something on the way to the office. Of course, don't stop for something of the donut or egg/muffin variety. You know what to do!

Do you wait too long before eating and then find yourself starving, so you reach for something high-fat or sugary? Maybe you're eating all your heaviest foods right before you hit the hay—this isn't a good idea. Try to change your patterns to allow for an earlier dinner. You might also want to rearrange your eating pattern by having your big meal at lunch and then eating lighter at dinner. Do whatever works best for you. Stop making excuses and fix it.

The next thing that I want you to examine is your *portion size*. This is where I am going to remind you to measure all your portions for a couple of days until you get the hang of what they should look like. You can eat more than one portion. Just be sure to make note of it, and be sure that it fits into your particular program. Almost all of us overestimate what our portions should be, but if you want to change your body, you've got to start paying closer attention.

Now I want you to examine your Dietary Recall to see *what is in your head* when you're eating. Look to see if you eat more when you're tired, because you don't have the energy to cook a healthful meal, and then figure out a way around it. Maybe you could clean and freeze some fish or chicken, then sauté it in stock with some frozen vegetables when you come home. Or do you find that you eat an entire box of fat-free cookies after a long conversation with your lover? Figure out what, if anything, sets you off, and try to work around it.

If you find yourself eating alone, do you allow yourself to eat more than if you have dinner with someone else? There is nothing wrong with eating alone except that some people use it as an excuse to eat more, and I don't want you to do that. Maybe you need to put the serving bowls or pots away before you start eating, so that you won't pick a few more mouthfuls out when you return to the kitchen with your dish.

We have to try to break ourselves of the habit that our parents have instilled by forcing us to finish every last scrap on our plates. Don't worry, no meal will be the last meal you get. Take comfort in the fact that you can always eat a little something later if you're still hungry. This brings back memories of me and my brothers licking our "choice" pieces of chicken or pie to be sure that someone else wouldn't grab it. It's a hard mentality to break. Instead, let's go back to Emily Post, where we find that it is polite to leave at least a little of each thing on your plate. This habit will save you lots of calories over time. And while we're at it, I'd like to scrap the "no-thank-you helping." If you don't want something, don't eat it. That is, unless it is something that you need to eat to maintain your balanced diet.

Where you are can impact your diet as well. Are you running from one place to another, with no time to stop and eat? Find a way to fit something healthful in. Take something with you. Get over the concept that all your meals should be hot—it's not necessary. If you have to go out for social or business reasons, maybe you can eat before you go out, and then just pick. Choose foods that don't have sauces or cheese that add lots of extra fat. Snack on pretzels at a party rather than Fritos or peanuts. Go out with a plan in your head. Solve the problem before you face it.

HOW TO SET GOALS

Weight loss should not be your major objective during this program. You might need to drop a few pant sizes, or chisel your muscles to greater definition, but who really cares what you *weigh*? It's just a number. Lose the fat. Change the way you eat. It's almost a guarantee that a side effect of the accomplishment of these goals will be weight loss.

I want to re-create the way you eat by introducing subtle changes that you can live with. Don't think about crazy diets ever again. You've been following the wrong game plan and it's time to redraw the plan.

On Peak 10, we set weekly goals and give ourselves weekly rewards. The goals should be easy, like to eat breakfast every day. We've learned how important breakfast is to our metabolism. Or aim to do the extra-credit "just abs" workout (page 139) three times a week. Aim to walk three miles each day. Rewards can include buying yourself a new piece of clothing, a CD, or tickets to a movie, giving yourself an extra half hour of sleep, watching your favorite TV show.

Your long-term goals should also be personal: to lower your cholesterol 20 points, to lose 5 percent body fat, to be able to run two miles, to be able to fit into your old jeans. Do the things that a lean person would do: go to the beach, order soup and a salad, go outside, ride a bike. Start to think like a lean, fit, healthy person. By setting these kinds of achievable, significant goals, you'll see noticeable differences in your body.

The program is designed so that you won't overtrain or burn out. You'll create a balance in your life. Your metabolism will go up. Looking in the mirror will be an inspiration to you. This is a progressive, goal-oriented program that involves all three of the components of fitness. The more you can put into it, the more you'll get out of it. At the end you'll say, "I don't want to go back to my old life."

I bet you still want to lose weight, so never let anyone say I didn't do you a favor. I know you're still getting on the scale. I know you still want to lose weight. So if that's what you want, I can help you set a realistic, specific weight-loss target based on how much of your weight should be lean muscle mass and how much should be fat.

First, multiply your weight by your body-fat percentage (which you determined on pages 23–24). Then subtract that number from your weight. For example: If a woman weighs 135 pounds and has a body-fat percentage of 24, then she has 32.4 pounds of fat (135 × .24 = 32.4) and 102 pounds of lean muscle mass (135 − 32.4 = 102). Therefore, 102 pounds of this woman's weight is *not* fat. This is her lean muscle mass (LMM).

Now, we all need some fat on our bodies. A healthful amount of fat for women is between 18 and 22 percent; for men, between 8 and 12 percent. We can determine your optimum weight using your current LMM. To find the *range* of weight that is safe for you, follow this equation. For women, divide your LMM by .82 and .78 to determine the high and the low ends of your low-fat weight range. For men, divide your LMM by .92 and .88 for your range. For example:

$$102 \div .82 = \mathbf{124}$$
$$102 \div .78 = \mathbf{131}$$

Although this 135-pound woman says that she wants to lose 15 pounds, a better goal would be to lose between 4 and 11 pounds of fat while maintaining (or increasing) the amount of muscle in her body. It's a much easier, safer goal than simply going on a diet.

So your goal is to decrease your fat weight while increasing your lean muscle mass. By aiming to change both your body-fat percentage *and* your weight ("I want to be 120 pounds!") you can set a realistic, attainable goal. And you'll look great.

CHOOSING THE CORRECT SHOES

Although walking and lifting weights are activities that our bodies were built to do, science has found ways to help us. With the right shoes we can reduce our risks of strain and injury. I've seen several clients start out on an aggressive walking program only to experience premature fatigue from worn-out running shoes. (They do get worn-out!)

Now, before a client and I go out for our first walk, I take him or her to a good sporting goods store and we pick out a new pair of sneakers. Peak 10 is going to be on the top of your list for the next ten weeks. You're going to rely on your feet a lot in the near future. Treat them right.

To buy the best pair of shoes for your feet, go to a store that specializes in athletic footwear. That way the salesperson will have some background in fitting shoes correctly.

Next, tell the salesperson specifics about your foot and your step. Do you have high arches? (If you step in water and then make a footprint, can you only see the ball and heel of your step?) Do you have flat feet? (If you step in water and then make a footprint, can you see your entire foot in the step?) Do your heels turn in when you walk? Look at an old pair of sneakers or shoes. Is the inside of the heel worn in? That means your feet are everted. If your shoes are worn down on the outside part of the heel, that means that your feet are inverted. Ask the salesperson for shoes that will help correct these problems.

Always go shopping for shoes (all kinds) at the end of the day, when you've been on your feet all day, because they might expand as the day goes on. When trying on shoes, wear the type of socks that you plan to exercise in. Avoid 100 percent cotton socks, which can cause blisters. There are some great thick socks on the market that are designed to absorb impact and limit blistering (Thorlo makes a great one). If the shoes pinch at all, don't buy them. Sneakers don't need to be "broken in." Don't let anyone tell you they do.

If you play a sport more than three times a week, then you need a sports-specific shoe. Although there are numerous "walking" shoes on the market, I recommend that you buy a *running* shoe, even if you plan to walk. They're not pretty, but they provide the best support—and you're going to need it.

HIGH-IMPACT WARNING

- Use Vaseline to reduce friction on feet or other body parts that rub and develop blisters from walking or running.
- High-intensity exercise can be hell on a woman's breasts if they are not properly supported. Always wear an exercise bra if you need one.
- Men should wear an athletic supporter or tight running gear for high-impact activities.

If You Get Injured

Injuries probably won't happen if you're careful and follow my guidance. Walking and lifting light weights are two safe forms of exercise. Very safe. But, of course, things happen. Here are things to look out for:

- Any sharp pain that happens while you're working out
- A feeling of ripping or tearing within your muscles
- An overwhelming feeling of breathlessness
- Dizziness

If something hurts suddenly, stop what you're doing right away. The best immediate solution for most injuries is called RICE, which stands for Rest, Ice, Compression, and Elevation. In other words, if you have an injury: rest, put ice on it, wrap it tight with a bandage (but not too tight), and raise it high (on a pillow, for example). If it is painful or feels unusual, or if your discomfort lasts for more than two days, see your doctor.

Staying on the Program

Don't underestimate the difficulty of doing a program, any program, whether it's Peak 10 or learning to ride a horse, without a coach. A coach will ask questions: How are you? What did you eat today? How fast are you running now? How much can you lift today? What are you aiming for? I ask such questions for several reasons: It helps me figure out my program for you, and it helps me show you how well you're doing later. It's also just because I care and I want to know. I want to know you, and you should want to know yourself. If you're afraid of finding out an answer, deal with that issue, but find out the answer anyway.

A coach creates a map for you to reach your goals. You have a starting point and a goal now. How are you going to get through the journey? I can help you.

I'll keep you pumped. That's one of the most important parts of my job. I'm not here to keep you angry at the diet industry or to keep you feeling scared that you'll never lose the weight. I'm here to keep you excited about your workout and your body. I have to tell you why we're doing extra crunches so that you'll *want* to do them. Not only because it keeps you coming back to me but because your body and your mind are not separate. If you tell yourself it's helping you and you enjoy doing it, you'll come back, you'll see the results, and we'll both be proud. Then I get to pat you on the back. And if I'm not there to do it, I want you to find someone else to do it, or do it yourself.

Now let's get started on the program.

8 Daily Logs:

Weeks One Through Three

BASE CAMP: WEEK ONE, DAY ONE   DATE: _____

DAILY NOTICE: Take your first measurements today.

This is the first day of your Peak 10 program. Before you begin, be sure to take your measurements. Always measure *before* you work out, because this is when your body is in its normal, natural state. Taking measurements after a workout may skew your results. Make sure at this time you have determined your Target Training Zone (see chapter 5) to maximize the aerobic portion of the program.

In starting this program, you are embarking on a real-life adventure. Along with the anticipation of a lean, toned, healthy body, many of my clients are often a bit nervous. This is a very normal and expected reaction. Remember that you are making positive changes in the way you look and feel. Just take my hand and follow my lead. Focus on all your body's functions. Your breathing, your heart rate, how your muscles feel. Become familiar with these new feelings. Should you feel any abnormal pain or discomfort, stop and consult with your physician.

Whether exercise is new to you or you've been active all along, stay with the prescribed program. Using the fat-burning segment of the workout as a warm-up will prepare you for your total body workout. Take time to stretch before and after each workout.

Take it slow the first few times through the Base Camp workout. Give yourself enough time to fully understand the mechanics of each exercise. I've left some space for you to record your recovery time. Your goal is to perform each exercise with perfect form to failure, then rest and start the next exercise, continuing down the list I have provided below. The recovery time should be long enough to catch your breath and get some strength back, so, the shorter the recovery time, the higher the intensity. Good luck!

Aerobic Activity	Activity	Warm-up	Core	Cool-down
Fat Burner/Warm-up		5 min.	15 min.	5 min.

Pre/Post Workout Stretch
Neck Stretch
Chest/Biceps
Shoulder/Upper Back
Modified Hurdler Stretch
Flat Back Hamstring (toe flexed)
Double Knee to Chest
Side Quad Stretch
Child Stretch
Calf Stretch

Perform one set of each to failure.

Toning Exercises	Reps	Recovery
1 Leg Extension	_____	_____ sec.
2 Leg Curl	_____	_____ sec.
3 Plié	_____	_____ sec.
4 Chest Press	_____	_____ sec.
5 Chest Fly	_____	_____ sec.
6 Bent-Over Row	_____	_____ sec.
7 Upright Row	_____	_____ sec.
8 Lateral Raise	_____	_____ sec.
9 Biceps Curl	_____	_____ sec.
10 Triceps Extension	_____	_____ sec.
11 Abdominal Crunch	_____	_____ sec.
12 Prone Hyperextension #1	_____	_____ sec.

BASE CAMP: WEEK ONE, DAY TWO   DATE: _____

DAILY NOTICE: Simple "fat burning" workout today. Use music to help motivate you.

Today's focus is on burning that stored fat beneath your skin. In order to condition your body to utilize fat as a major energy source, it's critical to start off slow. Choose an activity that you really enjoy and one that allows you complete control over the intensity (e.g., walking, stationary bike, stair climbing, treadmill). I always recommend walking. It is the activity that everyone can do, speeding up or slowing down when needed.

Refer to your personal training zones that we determined in chapter 5. Stay in each zone for the prescribed durations. It is in these first few weeks that you will become more aware of how your body reacts to exercise. This is why it is so important to keep all of your exercise very controlled. I've left space below for you to take notes of how you feel through each phase. Remember to breathe and to slow down when needed. Fat needs oxygen to burn, and if you're huffing and puffing, you're probably not burning much fat. My motto is, *moderate and steady wins the race.*

I know that you have a lot of information to try to assimilate all at once, but there's one more part of the program that I want to remind you about, and that is nutrition. If you don't follow a sensible diet, all the aerobic exercise in the world won't help you lose body fat. So please pay attention and stick to the program!

Aerobic Activity	Activity	Warm-up	Core	Cool-down
Fat Burner/Warm-up		10 min.	20 min.	5 min.

Pre/Post Workout Stretch
Neck Stretch
Chest/Biceps
Shoulder/Upper Back
Modified Hurdler Stretch
Flat Back Hamstring (toe flexed)
Double Knee to Chest
Side Quad Stretch
Child Stretch
Calf Stretch

NOTES: _____

_____

_____

_____

_____

BASE CAMP: WEEK ONE, DAY THREE   DATE: _____

DAILY NOTICE: Focus on "mechanics of motion."

After warming up and stretching out, you are ready to begin your second day of the Base Camp workout. In order for you to maximize your results throughout this program, you need to train with perfect form, reaching the point of momentary muscular failure. Reaching failure is the easy part. It's the perfect form that is hard to maintain.

Start with little or no weight, move slowly through each exercise. Feel the muscle contract and relax through each repetition. In the beginning it may be difficult to isolate the muscle or muscle group that you are working. It is also common to feel discomfort in a completely different muscle altogether. Over time and with proper form and mechanics you will better focus on the areas that you are working.

Some people have a low energy level just after they start a new program. If you start off real strong and feel weak today, don't be discouraged. Just do what you can and get through your workout. Your energy level will increase again in the next few days and you'll be back on track. Just be sure not to use this slump as a reason to stop the program.

You might notice an increase in your appetite. This is normal when you increase your activity level. Take the time to plan out your daily menu during these first few weeks to be sure that you stick to the plan. You can do it!

AEROBIC ACTIVITY	ACTIVITY	WARM-UP	CORE	COOL-DOWN
Fat Burner/Warm-up		5 min.	15 min.	5 min.

PRE/POST WORKOUT STRETCH	TONING EXERCISES	REPS	RECOVERY
Neck Stretch	1 Leg Extension	_____	_____ sec.
Chest/Biceps	2 Leg Curl	_____	_____ sec.
Shoulder/Upper Back	3 Plié	_____	_____ sec.
Modified Hurdler Stretch	4 Chest Press	_____	_____ sec.
Flat Back Hamstring (toe flexed)	5 Chest Fly	_____	_____ sec.
	6 Bent-Over Row	_____	_____ sec.
Double Knee to Chest	7 Upright Row	_____	_____ sec.
Side Quad Stretch	8 Lateral Raise	_____	_____ sec.
Child Stretch	9 Biceps Curl	_____	_____ sec.
Calf Stretch	10 Triceps Extension	_____	_____ sec.
	11 Abdominal Crunch	_____	_____ sec.
	12 Prone Hyperextension #1	_____	_____ sec.

BASE CAMP: WEEK ONE, DAY FOUR   DATE: _____

DAILY NOTICE: Take today off and rest. Great job!!

While on the Peak 10 program, rest is a much needed and required component. It is as important as the workout and shouldn't be overlooked. Many individuals have a hard time slowing down once they get going in the program. Just because I ask you to rest doesn't mean that you're not on the program.

You still need to stick to your nutritional guidelines. Watch your food portions to prevent backsliding on your days off. If you have extra time today, chop some fresh veggies as snacks for the next week.

This is a great time to reevaluate what you have accomplished over the past few days. Update your notes and Dietary Recall. How is the routine working in your schedule? Make the needed modifications to fit it all in. Stay organized and plan out the rest of the week. You're doing a terrific job. It's *your* body—you *deserve* all the attention.

BASE CAMP: WEEK ONE, DAY FIVE   DATE: _____

DAILY NOTICE: Burn fat, burn calories.

In combining resistance training with aerobic conditioning, you are swinging a double-edged sword. Weight training increases lean muscle, which requires more energy (fat) to function. By increasing your activity through aerobic exercise with more lean muscle, you are burning even more stored fat.

I'll tell *you* what I tell my clients: "Let's get out there and empty those fuel tanks and lean it out."

Don't forget to drink plenty of water. It might take a while to get accustomed to the increased fluid consumption, so get on it.

AEROBIC ACTIVITY	ACTIVITY	WARM-UP	CORE	COOL-DOWN
Fat Burner/Warm-up		10 min.	20 min.	5 min.

PRE/POST WORKOUT STRETCH
Neck Stretch
Chest/Biceps
Shoulder/Upper Back
Modified Hurdler Stretch
Flat Back Hamstring (toe flexed)
Double Knee to Chest
Side Quad Stretch
Child Stretch
Calf Stretch

NOTES: _____

_____

_____

_____

_____

_____

_____

_____

BASE CAMP: WEEK ONE, DAY SIX DATE: _____

DAILY NOTICE: Determine the right weight for the job.

After warming up and stretching out, you are ready to begin your third day of the Base Camp workout. Like the other two, continue to focus on form. You might already notice your recovery time beginning to lessen. You might even feel stronger and might need to increase your resistance in certain exercises. Remember to move slow and controlled through each repetition.

When it applies, select a weight that allows you to reach momentary muscular failure somewhere between 15 and 20 reps. If you're having trouble reaching 15, lighten up the weight and do additional repetitions. On the other hand, if you're completing more than 20, try to increase the weight a little and push to failure.

Again, it's reaching failure that has the greatest impact on changing your body. Keep your movement smooth and flowing and concentrate on achieving perfect form.

With perfect form and pushing through to failure you're on your way to a stronger, more toned, fat-burning body.

AEROBIC ACTIVITY	ACTIVITY	WARM-UP	CORE	COOL-DOWN
Fat Burner/Warm-up		5 min.	15 min.	5 min.

PRE/POST WORKOUT STRETCH	TONING EXERCISES	REPS	RECOVERY
Neck Stretch	1 Leg Extension	_____	_____ sec.
Chest/Biceps	2 Leg Curl	_____	_____ sec.
Shoulder/Upper Back	3 Plié	_____	_____ sec.
Modified Hurdler Stretch	4 Chest Press	_____	_____ sec.
	5 Chest Fly	_____	_____ sec.
Flat Back Hamstring (toe flexed)	6 Bent-Over Row	_____	_____ sec.
Double Knee to Chest	7 Upright Row	_____	_____ sec.
Side Quad Stretch	8 Lateral Raise	_____	_____ sec.
Child Stretch	9 Biceps Curl	_____	_____ sec.
Calf Stretch	10 Triceps Extension	_____	_____ sec.
	11 Abdominal Crunch	_____	_____ sec.
	12 Prone Hyperextension #1	_____	_____ sec.

BASE CAMP: WEEK ONE, DAY SEVEN   DATE: _____

DAILY NOTICE: End of week one, way to go!!

Good job! You've made it through the first week. You'll get stronger and feel better each week. Enjoy your day off.

NOTES: _____

_____

_____

_____

_____

_____

_____

_____

_____

Base Camp: Week Two, Day One

DAILY NOTICE: Total body workout with emphasis on lower body.

After you warm up and stretch, today's workout will be the same but with a little twist. Try moving through the first four exercises with less than 60 seconds of rest between each exercise. This will boost the intensity, encouraging you to work a little harder. The reason for this is to help you increase your muscular endurance. With increased muscular endurance, your regular daily activities will begin to seem effortless.

Try one of the heartier snacks today if you need the extra energy. Are you eating the proper ratio of protein, carbs, and fat?

Start this week off right and get another great workout in. Every day you get that much closer to the top.

Aerobic Activity	Activity	Warm-up	Core	Cool-down
Fat Burner/Warm-up		5 min.	15 min.	5 min.

Pre/Post Workout Stretch	Toning Exercises	Reps	Recovery
Neck Stretch	1 Leg Extension	_____	_____ sec.
Chest/Biceps	2 Leg Curl	_____	_____ sec.
Shoulder/Upper Back	3 Plié	_____	_____ sec.
Modified Hurdler Stretch	4 Chest Press	_____	_____ sec.
Flat Back Hamstring (toe flexed)	5 Chest Fly	_____	_____ sec.
	6 Bent-Over Row	_____	_____ sec.
Double Knee to Chest	7 Upright Row	_____	_____ sec.
Side Quad Stretch	8 Lateral Raise	_____	_____ sec.
Child Stretch	9 Biceps Curl	_____	_____ sec.
Calf Stretch	10 Triceps Extension	_____	_____ sec.
	11 Abdominal Crunch	_____	_____ sec.
	12 Prone Hyperextension #1	_____	_____ sec.

DAILY NOTICE: Exercise helps to reduce stress.

Along with making you aesthetically better, exercise helps reduce some of your daily stress. Our bodies seem to store and carry stress very much like a sponge sucks up water. Some of us soak up less than others, but in general we all need a release valve and a walk, a run, or 35 minutes on your stationary bike or treadmill will generally do the trick.

Prepare yourself for your workout by eating something light an hour or more before you start (depending on your physiology, you might need more or less time to digest). Take the time to get into comfortable loose clothing and the appropriate shoes for the activity. Stretch out and start off slow. Take a few really deep cleansing breaths and be on your way. Enjoy this time. It doesn't have to be painful or unpleasant. You know your own fitness level. Stick with it and I'm sure that you will feel better every day.

Aerobic Activity	Activity	Warm-up	Core	Cool-down
Fat Burner/Warm-up		10 min.	20 min.	5 min.

Pre/Post Workout Stretch

Neck Stretch

Chest/Biceps

Shoulder/Upper Back

Modified Hurdler Stretch

Flat Back Hamstring (toe flexed)

Double Knee to Chest

Side Quad Stretch

Child Stretch

Calf Stretch

NOTES: _____

_____

_____

_____

_____

_____

_____

BASE CAMP: WEEK TWO, DAY THREE   DATE: _____

DAILY NOTICE: If you slip during the climb, you don't have to fall.

Repeat the same training prescription from day one of this week. Take a look at your training data from that day. Okay, impress me. Try to improve upon your results from the other day. In essence that's what this program is all about. You are building upon each day that came before. This is why consistency is so important.

While I'm on the subject of consistency, let's talk briefly about inconsistency. Should you run into a problem with scheduling, just pick up the workout from where you left off. This is not a Monday through Sunday workout plan. Yes, there are seven days in each week, but as long as you're moving forward, missing a scheduled session once in a while won't sabotage your results. But if you're serious about attaining the body you deserve, stick with it. Your program won't let you down.

Some people also experience a brief lapse in judgment involving food. If you fall off the nutritional track, don't be discouraged, and don't go further off because of a slip. Get back on track as soon as you can and you will limit your downside. But don't underestimate the importance of the nutritional component!

Aerobic Activity	Activity	Warm-up	Core	Cool-down
Fat Burner/Warm-up		5 min.	15 min.	5 min.

Pre/Post Workout Stretch	Toning Exercises	Reps	Recovery
Neck Stretch	1 Leg Extension	_____	_____ sec.
Chest/Biceps	2 Leg Curl	_____	_____ sec.
Shoulder/Upper Back	3 Plié	_____	_____ sec.
Modified Hurdler Stretch	4 Chest Press	_____	_____ sec.
Flat Back Hamstring (toe flexed)	5 Chest Fly	_____	_____ sec.
	6 Bent-Over Row	_____	_____ sec.
Double Knee to Chest	7 Upright Row	_____	_____ sec.
Side Quad Stretch	8 Lateral Raise	_____	_____ sec.
Child Stretch	9 Biceps Curl	_____	_____ sec.
Calf Stretch	10 Triceps Extension	_____	_____ sec.
	11 Abdominal Crunch	_____	_____ sec.
	12 Prone Hyperextension #1	_____	_____ sec.

Base Camp: Week Two, Day Four

DATE: _____

DAILY NOTICE: Rest up, you deserve it.

Today is another great day to devote to nutrition. If you find that you're not following the plan, you might want to begin writing down what you eat each day in a little notebook that you can carry with you wherever you go. This will help you see what you are doing wrong and then you can take steps to change. Think lean!

Base Camp: Week Two, Day Five

DATE: _____

DAILY NOTICE: Let's condition your heart and lungs.

Another day, another new adventure. Today's workout will focus on increasing cardio-respiratory capacity. In other words we will be increasing your heart rate and breathing to get your heart and lungs in better shape. "Why?" you ask. First of all, with a stronger, more efficient heart and lungs, you won't be sucking wind every time you climb up a flight of stairs. Secondly, it's all part of a complete package. You wouldn't want to own a beautiful sports car with a defunct engine, would you?

Cardio conditioning differs slightly from aerobic fat burning. Instead of moving at a moderate intensity after warming up, you will train with more intensity, closer to your Anaerobic Threshold. Remember, the Anaerobic Threshold is the point at which your body is not getting enough oxygen to burn fat for fuel. You tend to burn more carbohydrates at and above this level, but that's okay. Our objective here is to condition your heart and lungs, not to burn tons of fat. It's all part of building a well-balanced, strong, and healthy body.

Start again by warming up for 5 minutes. During the core you will boost your efforts to a point where your breathing becomes rapid, but you shouldn't be gasping. Maintain this level throughout the core segment, then cool down as usual to where your heart rate and breathing are back to normal.

Drink plenty of water before and after you exercise.

Aerobic Activity	Activity	Warm-up	Core	Cool-down
Cardio Conditioning		5 min.	10 min.	3 min.

Pre/Post Workout Stretch

Neck Stretch

Chest/Biceps

Shoulder/Upper Back

Modified Hurdler Stretch

Flat Back Hamstring (toe flexed)

Double Knee to Chest

Side Quad Stretch

Child Stretch

Calf Stretch

NOTES: _____

_____

_____

_____

_____

BASE CAMP: WEEK TWO, DAY SIX

DATE: _____

DAILY NOTICE: Wrapping up week two, finish strong.

After warming up and stretching out, let's get right into our strength and toning segment. Today we're going to train with less rest between exercises 1 through 6: that is, 60 seconds or less between exercises. If you can't keep up this pace, then continue at your own pace, and pick up the pace on your next strength-training day.

Remember to maintain the proper form throughout your workout, even though you are increasing the intensity. Great job, you're looking strong.

If you're ordering out for dinner, try some grilled fish without sauce and steamed veggies with vinegar or lemon. Finish it up with some decaf coffee or cappuccino.

AEROBIC ACTIVITY	ACTIVITY	WARM-UP	CORE	COOL-DOWN
Fat Burner/Warm-up		5 min.	15 min.	5 min.

PRE/POST WORKOUT STRETCH	TONING EXERCISES	REPS	RECOVERY
Neck Stretch	1 Leg Extension	_____	_____ sec.
Chest/Biceps	2 Leg Curl	_____	_____ sec.
Shoulder/Upper Back	3 Plié	_____	_____ sec.
Modified Hurdler Stretch	4 Chest Press	_____	_____ sec.
	5 Chest Fly	_____	_____ sec.
Flat Back Hamstring (toe flexed)	6 Bent-Over Row	_____	_____ sec.
Double Knee to Chest	7 Upright Row	_____	_____ sec.
Side Quad Stretch	8 Lateral Raise	_____	_____ sec.
Child Stretch	9 Biceps Curl	_____	_____ sec.
Calf Stretch	10 Triceps Extension	_____	_____ sec.
	11 Abdominal Crunch	_____	_____ sec.
	12 Prone Hyperextension #1	_____	_____ sec.

Base Camp: Week Two, Day Seven

DATE: _____

DAILY NOTICE: End of week two. Way to go!!

Remember to drink plenty of water and get the rest that your body needs. Spend some time working out your schedule for next week to be sure to fit it all in. Today is also a great day to try out a new recipe.

Before your next workout, remember it's time to measure again, so plan accordingly.

NOTES: _____

_____

_____

_____

_____

_____

_____

_____

_____

_____

_____

Base Camp: Week Three, Day One

DAILY NOTICE: Let's see how you measure up today . . .

First thing you need to do today is measure. Compare these measurements to your first measurements and see if there are any changes. If you've been following the program, you're probably starting to see some positive changes. If you don't see changes, don't be discouraged. Everyone is different and some people have to work longer before they realize changes. It's also a good idea to check your resting heart rate and adjust your training zones if your resting heart rate has changed.

If you are not making the progress that you would like, then your food intake is a great way to tweak it. Although it is important that you eat many times during the day, be sure to limit your portions. This is often where people encounter problems. Eating smaller portions will speed up your progress.

This is the last week at Base Camp, so let's get prepared for the Midway Ascent. This is a good week to catch up or move ahead. It is really important to start to fine-tune all three components of the program: diet, toning, and aerobic conditioning.

So let's get going. We're gonna boost up the duration of the fat-burning core, so that you'll burn more fat and better prepare yourself for the rest of the climb.

P.S. Don't forget to stretch before and after the workouts.

Aerobic Activity	Activity	Warm-up	Core	Cool-down
Fat Burner/Warm-up		10 min.	25 min.	5 min.

Pre/Post Workout Stretch
Neck Stretch
Chest/Biceps
Shoulder/Upper Back
Modified Hurdler Stretch
Flat Back Hamstring (toe flexed)
Double Knee to Chest
Side Quad Stretch
Child Stretch
Calf Stretch

BASE CAMP: WEEK THREE, DAY TWO   DATE: _____

DAILY NOTICE: Start your toning workout with cardio conditioning.

We're going to turn up the intensity today by adding the cardio conditioning to the Base Camp workout. You might need to take a few minutes between the two. Eating a piece of fruit or drinking a glass of fruit juice might be a good idea during the small break. You're going to need plenty of energy as you near the end of phase one of the program.

When you have settled down after the cardio conditioning, stretch and begin the strength and toning workout. Go at your own pace. Push to failure and, again, keep it slow and controlled.

You know the route, let's go!

AEROBIC ACTIVITY	ACTIVITY	WARM-UP	CORE	COOL-DOWN
Cardio Conditioning		5 min.	10 min.	3 min.

PRE/POST WORKOUT STRETCH	TONING EXERCISES	REPS	RECOVERY
Neck Stretch	1 Leg Extension	_____	_____ sec.
Chest/Biceps	2 Leg Curl	_____	_____ sec.
Shoulder/Upper Back	3 Plié	_____	_____ sec.
Modified Hurdler Stretch	4 Chest Press	_____	_____ sec.
	5 Chest Fly	_____	_____ sec.
Flat Back Hamstring (toe flexed)	6 Bent-Over Row	_____	_____ sec.
Double Knee to Chest	7 Upright Row	_____	_____ sec.
Side Quad Stretch	8 Lateral Raise	_____	_____ sec.
Child Stretch	9 Biceps Curl	_____	_____ sec.
Calf Stretch	10 Triceps Extension	_____	_____ sec.
	11 Abdominal Crunch	_____	_____ sec.
	12 Prone Hyperextension #1	_____	_____ sec.

BASE CAMP: WEEK THREE, DAY THREE   DATE: _____

DAILY NOTICE: Picking up the pace.

Take the time to have a healthful snack before you go to a party or meeting where they might be serving unhealthful food. If you're not starving when you get there, it will be easier to pass up the bad stuff.

Repeat day one of this week to continue to reduce the amount of stored body fat. If you find the fat-burning segment getting easy, try picking up the pace in the core. As your heart and lungs as well as your muscles get stronger, you will be able to cover longer distances over the same period of time. You are becoming more fit. That's great!

AEROBIC ACTIVITY	ACTIVITY	WARM-UP	CORE	COOL-DOWN
Fat Burner/Warm-up		10 min.	25 min.	5 min.

PRE/POST WORKOUT STRETCH
Neck Stretch
Chest/Biceps
Shoulder/Upper Back
Modified Hurdler Stretch
Flat Back Hamstring (toe flexed)
Double Knee to Chest
Side Quad Stretch
Child Stretch
Calf Stretch

DAILY NOTICE: It's heart, lungs, and abdominals today!

You will just be training your abdominals and midsection today. The cardio section will remain the same. With just abs to work out, you should really be able to push it out. It's important to stay extra focused when training your abdominals and lower back. Many individuals often feel pain when doing sit-ups and other midsection exercises. This often occurs when the exercise is done incorrectly. As always, discontinue exercising if you feel pain.

Take your time and work to failure during each exercise. As you have done with the other toning segments, track the number of repetitions you complete of each exercise. These numbers will become the basis for future achievements.

Work out smart and you will attain your goals. And don't forget: Calories do count. You need to limit them as well as fat intake to lose body fat. That's a great way to improve those abs. Do it!

AEROBIC ACTIVITY	ACTIVITY	WARM-UP	CORE	COOL-DOWN
Cardio Conditioning		5 min.	10 min.	3 min.

PRE/POST WORKOUT STRETCH	HOT SPOTS—JUST ABS	REPS	RECOVERY
Neck Stretch	1 Abdominal Crunch	_____	_____ sec.
Chest/Biceps	2 Side Crunch	_____	_____ sec.
Shoulder/Upper Back	3 Reverse Crunch	_____	_____ sec.
Modified Hurdler Stretch	4 Prone Hyperextension #2	_____	_____ sec.
Flat Back Hamstring (toe flexed)			
Double Knee to Chest			
Side Quad Stretch			
Child Stretch			
Calf Stretch			

BASE CAMP: WEEK THREE, DAY FIVE   DATE: _____

DAILY NOTICE: Rest up, you deserve it.

Remember that this schedule is just a guideline for when and how you should train. If you need to rearrange the days because of your schedule, just be sure to keep your workouts in order. But feel free to exchange rest days for workout days. For example, you might want to do tomorrow's workout today and then take tomorrow off.

If you enjoy pasta, try it with a basic tomato sauce. You can use a light coating of oil spray to sauté three cloves of garlic, add fresh basil, a can of stewed tomatoes, two tablespoons of tomato paste, and simmer for 1 hour. You can prepare a large pot and freeze it for convenience in the future. It is also great poured over some fresh seared tuna or chicken breast.

BASE CAMP: WEEK THREE, DAY SIX   DATE: _____

DAILY NOTICE: Finish strong.

After warming up and stretching out, you are ready to begin your last day of the Base Camp workout. You might even feel stronger and might need to increase your resistance in certain exercises. Remember to move slow and controlled through each repetition.

Again, select the appropriate weight that allows you to reach momentary muscular failure somewhere between 15 and 20 reps. If you're having trouble reaching 15, lighten up the weight and do additional repetitions. On the other hand, if you're completing more than 20, try to increase the weight a little and push to failure. Keep your movement smooth and flowing and concentrate on achieving perfect form.

The more familiar you become with the exercises, the greater the benefits. Keep up the intensity and always remain focused on form. You will really start to notice the physical changes taking place.

Remember that if you don't have junk food in your house, you're less likely to eat it. Besides, it isn't good for anyone else either. Enjoy your new healthier way of life.

AEROBIC ACTIVITY	ACTIVITY	WARM-UP	CORE	COOL-DOWN
Cardio Conditioning		5 min.	10 min.	3 min.

PRE/POST WORKOUT STRETCH	TONING EXERCISES	REPS	RECOVERY
Neck Stretch	1 Leg Extension	_____	_____ sec.
Chest/Biceps	2 Leg Curl	_____	_____ sec.
Shoulder/Upper Back	3 Plié	_____	_____ sec.
Modified Hurdler Stretch	4 Chest Press	_____	_____ sec.
	5 Chest Fly	_____	_____ sec.
Flat Back Hamstring (toe flexed)	6 Bent-Over Row	_____	_____ sec.
	7 Upright Row	_____	_____ sec.
Double Knee to Chest	8 Lateral Raise	_____	_____ sec.
Side Quad Stretch	9 Biceps Curl	_____	_____ sec.
Child Stretch	10 Triceps Extension	_____	_____ sec.
Calf Stretch	11 Abdominal Crunch	_____	_____ sec.
	12 Prone Hyperextension #1	_____	_____ sec.

BASE CAMP: WEEK THREE, DAY SEVEN   DATE: _____

DAILY NOTICE: End of week three. Congratulations!!

Rest and let your body recover from the exciting first three weeks of the Peak 10 program. Base Camp is behind us now and we are on our way to the Midway Ascent. This is an excellent time to take a look back on the climb. Pinpoint where your strengths and weaknesses are and plan on spending a little more time on the events that need to be polished.

Everything is moving along just perfectly. You're understanding how it fits together. You are figuring how to make the time to exercise. Plan, plan, and plan. Stay organized and prioritize.

The nutritional program stays the same, so you should be getting accustomed to your new eating patterns by now. Keep going and have fun!

NOTES: _____

_____

_____

_____

_____

_____

_____

_____

_____

_____

9 Daily Logs:

Weeks Four Through Seven

MIDWAY ASCENT: WEEK FOUR, DAY ONE

DATE: _____

DAILY NOTICE: Welcome to the Midway Ascent.

During our Midway Ascent, I will include additional exercises as well as modifications to the base of exercises that you have patiently become very familiar with. Take your time to learn and understand the mechanics of these additions and modifications. Refer back to the photos and descriptions in chapter 6.

You are moving up and improving physically every day. This workout might take more time to complete in the beginning, but after a while you will move through each day more and more efficiently. Take a look at the rest of the week ahead, set your schedule, and organize your time. In order to make the climb together, I need you with me every step of the way.

Don't forget to stretch before and after each workout. This is a great time to include a water break also. Are you "keeping it clear"?

AEROBIC ACTIVITY	ACTIVITY	WARM-UP	CORE	COOL-DOWN
Cardio Conditioning		5 min.	10 min.	3 min.

PRE/POST WORKOUT STRETCH	TONING EXERCISES	REPS	RECOVERY
Neck Stretch	1 Lunge **(New)**	_____	_____ sec.
Chest/Biceps	2 Leg Extension	_____	_____ sec.
Shoulder/Upper Back	3 Leg Curl	_____	_____ sec.
Modified Hurdler Stretch	4 Plié Slide (**Modified**)	_____	_____ sec.
Flat Back Hamstring (toe flexed)	5 Reverse Lunge **(New)**	_____	_____ sec.
	6 Outer Thigh **(New)**	_____	_____ sec.
Double Knee to Chest	7 Chest Press	_____	_____ sec.
Side Quad Stretch	8 Bent-Over Row	_____	_____ sec.
Child Stretch	9 Upright Row	_____	_____ sec.
Calf Stretch	10 Overhead Press **(New)**	_____	_____ sec.
	11 Biceps Curl	_____	_____ sec.
	12 Triceps Extension	_____	_____ sec.
	13 Abdominal Crunch	_____	_____ sec.
	14 Side Crunch **(New)**	_____	_____ sec.
	15 Reverse Crunch **(New)**	_____	_____ sec.
	16 Prone Hyperextension #2 (**Modified**)	_____	_____ sec.

MIDWAY ASCENT: WEEK FOUR, DAY TWO

DATE: _____

DAILY NOTICE: Burn fat in the "core."

Once again it's time to increase the duration of the fat-burning workout. I've been slowly upping the time that you spend in the core of the aerobic workout. At this point you have added 10 additional fat-burning minutes to this segment. Little by little you are making significant and lasting changes, not only burning fat but conditioning your body to use fat more often as a fuel source. You have identified your Optimum Fat Utilization Zone to maximize every step you take. Next time you feel like eating something unhealthful, remember that you have to work aerobically for approximately 10 to 15 minutes (in your core) for every 100 calories consumed.

Keep it burning!

AEROBIC ACTIVITY	ACTIVITY	WARM-UP	CORE	COOL-DOWN
Fat Burner/Warm-up		10 min.	30 min.	5 min.

PRE/POST WORKOUT STRETCH
Neck Stretch
Chest/Biceps
Shoulder/Upper Back
Modified Hurdler Stretch
Flat Back Hamstring (toe flexed)
Double Knee to Chest
Side Quad Stretch
Child Stretch
Calf Stretch

MIDWAY ASCENT: WEEK FOUR, DAY THREE

DAILY NOTICE: Day off. Check out Nanny Besio's Pasta e Fagioli (page 73).

Take advantage of these days off. Spend some extra time with family and friends. Let them know how you are doing and share with them a low-fat, highly nutritious, hearty meal. Try my mom's famous beans and macaroni. It's the best.

Midway Ascent: Week Four, Day Four

DATE: _____

DAILY NOTICE: Shoot to improve.

As you move through these early weeks of the program, you will be constantly challenged. One of your major goals throughout the program is to do better than you did in your last workout. Always remember that it's you against you. Compete with yourself and shoot for one rep more than you reached the last time.

When you challenge yourself, you will improve. Pack a healthful lunch to go.

Aerobic Activity	Activity	Warm-up	Core	Cool-down
Cardio Conditioning		5 min.	10 min.	3 min.

Pre/Post Workout Stretch	Toning Exercises	Reps	Recovery
Neck Stretch	1 Lunge	_____	_____ sec.
Chest/Biceps	2 Leg Extension	_____	_____ sec.
Shoulder/Upper Back	3 Leg Curl	_____	_____ sec.
Modified Hurdler Stretch	4 Plié Slide	_____	_____ sec.
	5 Reverse Lunge	_____	_____ sec.
Flat Back Hamstring (toe flexed)	6 Outer Thigh	_____	_____ sec.
Double Knee to Chest	7 Chest Press	_____	_____ sec.
Side Quad Stretch	8 Bent-Over Row	_____	_____ sec.
Child Stretch	9 Upright Row	_____	_____ sec.
Calf Stretch	10 Overhead Press	_____	_____ sec.
	11 Biceps Curl	_____	_____ sec.
	12 Triceps Extension	_____	_____ sec.
	13 Abdominal Crunch	_____	_____ sec.
	14 Side Crunch	_____	_____ sec.
	15 Reverse Crunch	_____	_____ sec.
	16 Prone Hyperextension #2	_____	_____ sec.

Midway Ascent: Week Four, Day Five

DATE: _____

DAILY NOTICE: Blaze a new trail today.

If you find that you are having trouble staying motivated, make a change. We are close to ending the fourth week of the program. Moving forward and upward means you are realizing changes in your body (increased endurance, reduced body fat, increased strength). Changing activities often helps maintain interest and keeps you challenged at the same time.

Keep on your nutritional program by adding some new recipes. There are tons of great recipe books out there. (See page 65 for some suggestions.)

When it comes to burning fat, moderate and steady does the trick. Keeping that philosophy in mind, try adding a new aerobic activity to your repertoire. Follow the same prescription. Include the warm-up, core, and cool-down. Continue to monitor your heart rate and pay close attention to your level of exertion. Remember, you need to breathe to burn fat.

Aerobic Activity	Activity	Warm-up	Core	Cool-down
Fat Burner/Warm-up		10 min.	30 min.	5 min.

Pre/Post Workout Stretch
Neck Stretch
Chest/Biceps
Shoulder/Upper Back
Modified Hurdler Stretch
Flat Back Hamstring (toe flexed)
Double Knee to Chest
Side Quad Stretch
Child Stretch
Calf Stretch

Midway Ascent: Week Four, Day Six

DATE: _____

DAILY NOTICE: Work those abs!

You will just be training your abdominals and midsection today. The cardio section will remain the same. With just abs to work out, you should really be able to push it out. It's important to stay extra focused when training your abdominals and lower back. Take your time and work to failure during each exercise. As you do with the other toning segments, track the number of repetitions you complete of each exercise.

In order to have beautifully defined abdominals, you must realize that doing a million sit-ups every day won't work if you're not limiting your fat intake and burning off the fat that often blankets these spectacular muscles. If you're following the program, you will soon be realizing the beauty that lies within.

Work out smart and you will attain your goals. Do it!

AEROBIC ACTIVITY	ACTIVITY	WARM-UP	CORE	COOL-DOWN
Cardio Conditioning		5 min.	10 min.	3 min.

PRE/POST WORKOUT STRETCH	HOT SPOTS—JUST ABS	REPS	RECOVERY
Neck Stretch	1 Abdominal Crunch	_____	_____ sec.
Chest/Biceps	2 Side Crunch	_____	_____ sec.
Shoulder/Upper Back	3 Reverse Crunch	_____	_____ sec.
Modified Hurdler Stretch	4 Prone Hyperextension #2	_____	_____ sec.
Flat Back Hamstring (toe flexed)			
Double Knee to Chest			
Side Quad Stretch			
Child Stretch			
Calf Stretch			

MIDWAY ASCENT: WEEK FOUR, DAY SEVEN

DATE: _____

DAILY NOTICE: Rest today and take time to reflect.

Take today off from training. As the weeks progress and you become more fit, you will find your energy levels increasing. This is one of the benefits of exercise and eating right. Take notice of how you feel and the difference exercise and proper nutrition can make in your life. You need to realize how much better you feel in order to continue your climb to peak physical condition.

DAILY NOTICE: It has been two weeks. Time to measure and compare.

At this point in the program changes are taking place every day. When taking measurements, try measuring twice, then take the average of your two measurements. Fill out the progress chart that I have provided in Appendix 1 in the back of the book. Also go back and recalculate your Target Training Zone. As you become more fit, your numbers might change.

If you find that you are falling short of your expectations, write down specifically what you want to achieve this week and for the weeks remaining. Along with writing down what you want, write down exactly what you will do to attain these goals (e.g., becoming more diligent in reducing fat and sugar intakes, making sure to complete each scheduled training day, etc.).

Remember, it is you who possess the secrets of a healthier, leaner, more fit body. With my help, you will achieve and attain your goals. Together, we will climb to the top of this mountain and appreciate how great it feels to be fit.

Follow the workout I have provided for you today and have a productive and healthful week.

Aerobic Activity	Activity	Warm-up	Core	Cool-down
Fat Burner/Warm-up		10 min.	30 min.	5 min.

Pre/Post Workout Stretch
Neck Stretch
Chest/Biceps
Shoulder/Upper Back
Modified Hurdler Stretch
Flat Back Hamstring (toe flexed)
Double Knee to Chest
Side Quad Stretch
Child Stretch
Calf Stretch

Midway Ascent: Week Five, Day Two

DAILY NOTICE: Stay focused and keep moving up.

Using cardio conditioning as your warm-up, move right into the Midway Ascent routine. Continue to practice and perfect the new additions and modifications that I have provided. As I've said, "It's not easy, but it's simple." Becoming more familiar with each exercise enables you to understand and master your every move. Plug in your desire and the motivation to be your very best and you will achieve your goals.

You know what you want. Together we have designed the plan to get you there. Don't stop till you reach the top.

P.S. Don't forget to stretch before and after each workout. Write down what you're eating if you begin to slip.

AEROBIC ACTIVITY	ACTIVITY	WARM-UP	CORE	COOL-DOWN
Cardio Conditioning		5 min.	10 min.	3 min.

PRE/POST WORKOUT STRETCH	TONING EXERCISES	REPS	RECOVERY
Neck Stretch	1 Lunge	_____	_____ sec.
Chest/Biceps	2 Leg Extension	_____	_____ sec.
Shoulder/Upper Back	3 Leg Curl	_____	_____ sec.
Modified Hurdler Stretch	4 Plié Slide	_____	_____ sec.
Flat Back Hamstring (toe flexed)	5 Reverse Lunge	_____	_____ sec.
	6 Outer Thigh	_____	_____ sec.
Double Knee to Chest	7 Chest Press	_____	_____ sec.
Side Quad Stretch	8 Bent-Over Row	_____	_____ sec.
Child Stretch	9 Upright Row	_____	_____ sec.
Calf Stretch	10 Overhead Press	_____	_____ sec.
	11 Biceps Curl	_____	_____ sec.
	12 Triceps Extension	_____	_____ sec.
	13 Abdominal Crunch	_____	_____ sec.
	14 Side Crunch	_____	_____ sec.
	15 Reverse Crunch	_____	_____ sec.
	16 Prone Hyperextension #2	_____	_____ sec.

Midway Ascent: Week Five, Day Three

DATE: _____

DAILY NOTICE: Rest and recover. No training today.

Treat yourself to a warm and relaxing bath. Allow your muscles the chance to regenerate. It is during the time you are resting, particularly sleeping, that your muscles and organs repair and rebuild. Make certain that you are giving your body the nutrients it needs as well as plenty of water to ensure hydration.

If at any time while on the program you come down with a cold, flu, or any common illness, take time off and then start up where you left off. If you are incapable of exercising for more than 10 days, repeat the week you completed last and move forward from there. Even though you can't exercise, you should always be eating low-fat, high-fiber meals. Eating this way will allow you to maintain all that you have worked for.

Midway Ascent: Week Five, Day Four DATE: _____

DAILY NOTICE: Lighten up in the warm-up and turn up the toning.

Start the workout today by doing your pretoning warm-up with lower intensity. This will allow for more energy in the toning segment of the workout. At this point in the Midway Ascent, you should be becoming more familiar with the new and modified exercises I have included. Try and challenge yourself by limiting your recovery time between each exercise. This will boost the intensity of the workout, encouraging your body to adapt to a higher level of conditioning.

High intensity, as far as you and I are concerned, is taking your training to a level higher than you have already been. Keep up a steady pace throughout the workout and rest enough to comfortably and safely move through and complete all the exercises below. Remember that pain is an indication to stop. Should you feel any pain or discomfort, stop and consult your physician.

Practicing perfect mechanics and maintaining smooth and steady movements throughout the exercises that I have prescribed will assure a highly productive, low-risk workout. Refer to chapter 6 for specific instructions and illustrations of all the exercises listed below.

Today might be a great day for a comfort meal of low-fat grilled cheese and soup. Keep up the good work!

Aerobic Activity	Activity	Warm-up	Core	Cool-down
Fat Burner/Warm-up		5 min.	15 min.	5 min.

PRE/POST WORKOUT STRETCH	TONING EXERCISES	REPS	RECOVERY
Neck Stretch	1 Lunge	_____	_____ sec.
Chest/Biceps	2 Leg Extension	_____	_____ sec.
Shoulder/Upper Back	3 Leg Curl	_____	_____ sec.
Modified Hurdler Stretch	4 Plié Slide	_____	_____ sec.
Flat Back Hamstring (toe flexed)	5 Reverse Lunge	_____	_____ sec.
	6 Outer Thigh	_____	_____ sec.
Double Knee to Chest	7 Chest Press	_____	_____ sec.
Side Quad Stretch	8 Bent-Over Row	_____	_____ sec.
Child Stretch	9 Upright Row	_____	_____ sec.
Calf Stretch	10 Overhead Press	_____	_____ sec.
	11 Biceps Curl	_____	_____ sec.
	12 Triceps Extension	_____	_____ sec.
	13 Abdominal Crunch	_____	_____ sec.
	14 Side Crunch	_____	_____ sec.
	15 Reverse Crunch	_____	_____ sec.
	16 Prone Hyperextension #2	_____	_____ sec.

DAILY NOTICE: Cover more distance in the same amount of time.

In training to burn fat you have to remember two important things: distance and duration. Whether you're walking, cycling, swimming, or stair climbing, you can boost the intensity by going further in the same amount of time. How do we do that? Move a little faster. By knowing how many miles, laps, or flights of stairs you cover over a set period of time, you have a goal to meet or beat.

Today, try to cover more distance during the core segment of the aerobic workout. Do this by training in the higher end of your Optimum Fat Utilization Zone. Should you feel that you are surpassing your Anaerobic Threshold, back off and settle back down to a more comfortable pace. Change the intensity gradually, giving your body a chance to adjust. Keep track of the distances you cover during all aerobic activity. Challenge yourself and slowly add more and more distance to each session. Remember, you don't need to break any world records, just do a little better each time. And please remember to drink plenty of water—your body really needs it.

AEROBIC ACTIVITY	ACTIVITY	WARM-UP	CORE	COOL-DOWN
Fat Burner/Warm-up		10 min.	30 min.	5 min.

PRE/POST WORKOUT STRETCH
Neck Stretch
Chest/Biceps
Shoulder/Upper Back
Modified Hurdler Stretch
Flat Back Hamstring (toe flexed)
Double Knee to Chest
Side Quad Stretch
Child Stretch
Calf Stretch

MIDWAY ASCENT: WEEK FIVE, DAY SIX

DAILY NOTICE: Rest up and eat right.

MIDWAY ASCENT: WEEK FIVE, DAY SEVEN

DATE: _____

DAILY NOTICE: No ifs, ands, or Butts!

You will just be focus-training your buttocks and thighs today. The cardio section will remain the same. With the emphasis on butt and thighs, you should really be able to push it out. Take your time and work to failure during each exercise. As with the other toning segments, track the number of repetitions you complete of each exercise to track your progress.

In order to attain a well-toned derrière, I have pulled some of my favorites out of the workout. If you understand the mechanics of the exercises, you will have no trouble moving right through each exercise. I have included an additional exercise that will really help isolate the buttocks, Heel-ups (see page 137).

Work out smart and you will attain your goals. Give yourself the boost that you deserve with an extra healthful snack today. Go to it!

AEROBIC ACTIVITY	ACTIVITY	WARM-UP	CORE	COOL-DOWN
Cardio Conditioning		5 min.	10 min.	3 min.

PRE/POST WORKOUT STRETCH	HOT SPOTS—JUST BUTT	REPS	RECOVERY
Neck Stretch	1 Lunge	_____	_____ sec.
Chest/Biceps	2 Leg Curl	_____	_____ sec.
Shoulder/Upper Back	3 Plié	_____	_____ sec.
Modified Hurdler Stretch	4 Reverse Lunge	_____	_____ sec.
Flat Back Hamstring (toe flexed)	5 Heel-ups (**New**)	_____	_____ sec.
Double Knee to Chest			
Side Quad Stretch			
Child Stretch			
Calf Stretch			

DAILY NOTICE: Take measurements and reevaluate.

If you've stuck with the program this far, you are seeing some incredible changes in your body. Congratulations, you look great. If you want to turn up the volume a little more, start a new Dietary Recall and continue to write down everything that you eat—and I mean everything. After a couple of days, you will see where your diet could use some improvement. Make the positive changes and move forward.

MIDWAY ASCENT: WEEK SIX, DAY TWO   DATE: _____

DAILY NOTICE: Increase cardio conditioning.

Simply add 2 additional minutes to the core segment of your cardio conditioning. Maintain steady and rhythmic intensity throughout the workout. Successfully complete the Midway Ascent workout and be sure to stretch slowly before and after the workout.

Are you eating enough fruit and vegetables? Remember that they are some of the best sources of vitamins, minerals, and especially fiber. Not getting enough fiber can really slow you down. Broccoli and apples are two of my favorites.

AEROBIC ACTIVITY	ACTIVITY	WARM-UP	CORE	COOL-DOWN
Cardio Conditioning		5 min.	12 min.	3 min.

PRE/POST WORKOUT STRETCH	TONING EXERCISES	REPS	RECOVERY
Neck Stretch	1 Lunge	_____	_____ sec.
Chest/Biceps	2 Leg Extension	_____	_____ sec.
Shoulder/Upper Back	3 Leg Curl	_____	_____ sec.
Modified Hurdler Stretch	4 Plié Slide	_____	_____ sec.
	5 Reverse Lunge	_____	_____ sec.
Flat Back Hamstring (toe flexed)	6 Outer Thigh	_____	_____ sec.
Double Knee to Chest	7 Chest Press	_____	_____ sec.
Side Quad Stretch	8 Bent-Over Row	_____	_____ sec.
Child Stretch	9 Upright Row	_____	_____ sec.
Calf Stretch	10 Overhead Press	_____	_____ sec.
	11 Biceps Curl	_____	_____ sec.
	12 Triceps Extension	_____	_____ sec.
	13 Abdominal Crunch	_____	_____ sec.
	14 Side Crunch	_____	_____ sec.
	15 Reverse Crunch	_____	_____ sec.
	16 Prone Hyperextension #2	_____	_____ sec.

Midway Ascent: Week Six, Day Three

DATE: _____

DAILY NOTICE: Take a walk.

Whatever your aerobic activity of choice may be, today I want you to ask a friend to take a nice relaxing walk. It's perfectly fine if the friend is of the four-legged variety. It is always nice to know that even a comfortable walk is considered exercise. Most people don't have any problem putting on some comfortable clothing and a pair of sneakers and stepping out to a local park. Walking with a friend or family member is a great way to introduce exercise to a loved one, and a great time to catch up on some friendly conversation.

Keep up the great new nutritional outlook. Don't let friends or relatives sabotage your efforts by enticing you with unhealthful foods . . . stay strong, you know what's best for you.

Aerobic Activity	Activity	Warm-up	Core	Cool-down
Fat Burner/Warm-up		5 min.	25+ min.	5 min.

Pre/Post Workout Stretch
Neck Stretch
Chest/Biceps
Shoulder/Upper Back
Modified Hurdler Stretch
Flat Back Hamstring (toe flexed)
Double Knee to Chest
Side Quad Stretch
Child Stretch
Calf Stretch

Midway Ascent: Week Six, Day Four   DATE: _____

DAILY NOTICE: Just arms!

You will just be focus-training your arms today. The cardio section will remain the same with the emphasis on biceps and triceps. Take your time and work to failure during each exercise. As with the other toning segments, track the number of repetitions you complete of each exercise. These numbers will become the basis for future achievements.

In order to attain well-toned arms, I have pulled out some of my favorites. Understand the mechanics of the exercises and you will have no trouble moving right through the series. I have included an additional exercise that will really help isolate the back of your upper arms, or triceps, the Triceps Dip (see page 138).

Work out smart and you will attain your goals. Do it!

Are you getting enough calcium? Some of the best sources of calcium and protein are nonfat yogurt and cottage cheese. Try some balsamic vinegar on the cottage cheese, or pour the yogurt over some chopped fresh fruit . . . you'll love it.

Aerobic Activity	Activity	Warm-up	Core	Cool-down
Cardio Conditioning		5 min.	12 min.	3 min.

Pre/Post Workout Stretch	Hot Spots—Just Arms	Reps	Recovery
Neck Stretch	1 Biceps Curl	_____	_____ sec.
Chest/Biceps	2 Triceps Extension	_____	_____ sec.
Shoulder/Upper Back	3 Triceps Dip (**New**)	_____	_____ sec.
Modified Hurdler Stretch			
Flat Back Hamstring (toe flexed)			
Double Knee to Chest			
Side Quad Stretch			
Child Stretch			
Calf Stretch			

Midway Ascent: Week Six, Day Five DATE: _____

DAILY NOTICE: Rest and recover. No training today.

Rest, relax, and recover.

Throw a chicken in the oven so that you can make chicken salads or sandwiches for the next few days. It's healthful and simple.

Midway Ascent: Week Six, Day Six DATE: _____

DAILY NOTICE: Longest fat burner so far.

All 55 minutes of today's workout will be dedicated to burning calories. Remember, you need to create a caloric deficit by means of limited caloric intake and increased caloric expenditure. You are in the process of permanent modification. Running on a deficit is not our goal. We want to maintain a body that is lean and strong as opposed to fat and weak. Our goal is to learn and understand the principles of a healthier life and continue to practice these principles long after the program is over.

Aerobic Activity	Activity	Warm-up	Core	Cool-down
Fat Burner/Warm-up		10 min.	40 min.	5 min.
Pre/Post Workout Stretch				
Neck Stretch				
Chest/Biceps				
Shoulder/Upper Back				
Modified Hurdler Stretch				
Flat Back Hamstring (toe flexed)				
Double Knee to Chest				
Side Quad Stretch				
Child Stretch				
Calf Stretch				

MIDWAY ASCENT: WEEK SIX, DAY SEVEN

DATE: _____

DAILY NOTICE: Four exercises, recover and continue.

After a brief warm-up, stretch and prepare for your workout. Today we will be moving through the Midway Ascent with little rest between every four exercises. Take as long as you need to catch your breath and let your heart rate return to its normal resting level. After this recovery period continue through the workout.

Maintain perfect form and push to momentary muscular failure.

Don't forget to stretch before and after every workout. And keep drinking that water!

AEROBIC ACTIVITY	ACTIVITY	WARM-UP	CORE	COOL-DOWN
Fat Burner/Warm-up		5 min.	15 min.	5 min.

PRE/POST WORKOUT STRETCH	TONING EXERCISES	REPS	RECOVERY
Neck Stretch	1 Lunge	_____	_____ sec.
Chest/Biceps	2 Leg Extension	_____	_____ sec.
Shoulder/Upper Back	3 Leg Curl	_____	_____ sec.
Modified Hurdler Stretch	4 Plié Slide	_____	_____ sec.
	5 Reverse Lunge	_____	_____ sec.
Flat Back Hamstring (toe flexed)	6 Outer Thigh	_____	_____ sec.
Double Knee to Chest	7 Chest Press	_____	_____ sec.
Side Quad Stretch	8 Bent-Over Row	_____	_____ sec.
Child Stretch	9 Upright Row	_____	_____ sec.
Calf Stretch	10 Overhead Press	_____	_____ sec.
	11 Biceps Curl	_____	_____ sec.
	12 Triceps Extension	_____	_____ sec.
	13 Abdominal Crunch	_____	_____ sec.
	14 Side Crunch	_____	_____ sec.
	15 Reverse Crunch	_____	_____ sec.
	16 Prone Hyperextension #2	_____	_____ sec.

MIDWAY ASCENT: WEEK SEVEN, DAY ONE

DATE: _____

DAILY NOTICE: Chart your progress and measure today.

Before you begin your fat-burning aerobic workout, take and chart your current measurements. This is our last week at the Midway Ascent. You have made significant changes in life, gaining control and harnessing your abilities to be your best. Continue to strive for your personal goals, making modifications where needed. Also take the time to recalculate your Target Training Zone. It might have changed as you have changed.

Changing your lifestyle in a positive way is the only means to successfully change the way you look and feel. If we follow a pattern that promotes a lean, strong, and healthy body, eventually that is what we will attain. Whether it be ten weeks or ten months, living a life of good nutrition and regular exercise will yield a healthier, more fit body.

On that note, stretch out and get that body working, and remember, "you are what you eat."

AEROBIC ACTIVITY	ACTIVITY	WARM-UP	CORE	COOL-DOWN
Fat Burner/Warm-up		10 min.	30 min.	5 min.

PRE/POST WORKOUT STRETCH

Neck Stretch

Chest/Biceps

Shoulder/Upper Back

Modified Hurdler Stretch

Flat Back Hamstring (toe flexed)

Double Knee to Chest

Side Quad Stretch

Child Stretch

Calf Stretch

Midway Ascent: Week Seven, Day Two

DATE: _____

DAILY NOTICE: Hot Spot!

Boost the cardio section up to 25 minutes total. Adjust your intensity to stay below your Anaerobic Threshold. Cool down and get focused on the "just butt" workout. You can continue to refer back to chapter 6 for the proper mechanics and form of the exercises. Push to improve your form and add additional repetitions for maximum results. Add or subtract from the supplemental resistance to reach failure between 15 and 20 reps.

The best prescription for a great butt is to reduce your body fat and tone it up. Nutrition is so important for the results of your program. Remember to stay on track. Each time you pass up something unhealthful, you will be that much better off in the long haul. Great job!

AEROBIC ACTIVITY	ACTIVITY	WARM-UP	CORE	COOL-DOWN
Cardio Conditioning		**5 min.**	**15 min.**	**5 min.**

PRE/POST WORKOUT STRETCH	HOT SPOTS—JUST BUTT	REPS	RECOVERY
Neck Stretch	1 Lunge	_____	_____ sec.
Chest/Biceps	2 Leg Curl	_____	_____ sec.
Shoulder/Upper Back	3 Plié	_____	_____ sec.
Modified Hurdler Stretch	4 Reverse Lunge	_____	_____ sec.
Flat Back Hamstring (toe flexed)	5 Heel-ups	_____	_____ sec.
Double Knee to Chest			
Side Quad Stretch			
Child Stretch			
Calf Stretch			

MIDWAY ASCENT: WEEK SEVEN, DAY THREE

DAILY NOTICE: Think fit to be fit. Rest today.

When you look in the mirror, what do you see? In order to live a life of good health and well-being, you need to think of yourself as a work in progress. You have the ability to be your physical best. You must believe that no matter where you are now, ultimately you will reach the top. Your peak!

MIDWAY ASCENT: WEEK SEVEN, DAY FOUR

DATE: _____

DAILY NOTICE: This is a great day to tone up those arms!

The workout today will include a 45-minute fat burner with a concentrated arm workout. Real simple and straight to the point. Continue on the path to a leaner, more toned body. Remember that the goal is to be your best. Each day that passes brings another day to improve.

Try Chris's Easy Dip today (page 49). It's great with fresh vegetables or a few pretzels. You will achieve your goals when you act upon your desires.

AEROBIC ACTIVITY	ACTIVITY	WARM-UP	CORE	COOL-DOWN
Fat Burner/Warm-up		10 min.	30 min.	5 min.

PRE/POST WORKOUT STRETCH	HOT SPOTS—JUST ARMS	REPS	RECOVERY
Neck Stretch	1 Biceps Curl	_____	_____ sec.
Chest/Biceps	2 Triceps Extension	_____	_____ sec.
Shoulder/Upper Back	3 Triceps Dip	_____	_____ sec.
Modified Hurdler Stretch			
Flat Back Hamstring (toe flexed)			
Double Knee to Chest			
Side Quad Stretch			
Child Stretch			
Calf Stretch			

MIDWAY ASCENT: WEEK SEVEN, DAY FIVE

DATE: _____

DAILY NOTICE: Burn fat and work those abs!

As in day four of this week, we will be spending more time on fat-burning aerobics. Along with the aerobic component, we will train abdominals after you have cooled down. With just abs to work out, you should really be able to push it out. Remember, it's important to stay extra focused when training your abdominals and lower back. Take your time and work to failure during each exercise.

The combination of these two workouts is just what the doctor ordered for lean and toned abdominals.

Today is a great day to keep track of your caloric intake and compare it to the daily intake that you calculated in chapter 4. Are you still on track? Make adjustments to your food habits to compensate for any discrepancies. Keep it up, you're doing a great job.

AEROBIC ACTIVITY	ACTIVITY	WARM-UP	CORE	COOL-DOWN
Fat Burner/Warm-up		10 min.	30 min.	5 min.

PRE/POST WORKOUT STRETCH	HOT SPOTS—JUST ABS	REPS	RECOVERY
Neck Stretch	1 Abdominal Crunch	_____	_____ sec.
Chest/Biceps	2 Side Crunch	_____	_____ sec.
Shoulder/Upper Back	3 Reverse Crunch	_____	_____ sec.
Modified Hurdler Stretch	4 Prone Hyperextension #2	_____	_____ sec.
Flat Back Hamstring (toe flexed)			
Double Knee to Chest			
Side Quad Stretch			
Child Stretch			
Calf Stretch			

MIDWAY ASCENT: WEEK SEVEN, DAY SIX

DAILY NOTICE: Take the day off from training today!

Just remember that a day off is not a day off of the nutritional program. You need to keep following that each day. By now you should be accustomed to your new pattern of eating. Enjoy the new easier feeling of healthful eating. This new eating style will help you to keep getting more and more trim as you grow older, rather than hanging on to extra pounds.

Midway Ascent: Week Seven, Day Seven

DATE: _____

DAILY NOTICE: Last day at the Midway Ascent!

Reduce your cardio-conditioning duration today and conserve your energy for a juiced-up Midway Ascent workout. Today is not only the last day of the week but the last day at the Midway Ascent. After warming up and stretching out, plan to complete four exercises with little or no rest. As you know, this will boost the intensity of the workout and help to create a higher level of adaptation. That means you will get more fit.

Keep the form and mechanics perfect. Keep this book close by so you can refer to the exercise descriptions in chapter 6 should you need to refresh your memory. Remember that I am here to help you succeed and show you the right path to the top.

Prepare yourself in advance for a possible boost in appetite by planning your next four days of food in advance. If you know what you're going to eat, your chances of making a bad food choice are reduced.

Aerobic Activity	Activity	Warm-up	Core	Cool-down
Cardio Conditioning		5 min.	12 min.	3 min.

Pre/Post Workout Stretch	Toning Exercises	Reps	Recovery
Neck Stretch	1 Lunge	_____	_____ sec.
Chest/Biceps	2 Leg Extension	_____	_____ sec.
Shoulder/Upper Back	3 Leg Curl	_____	_____ sec.
Modified Hurdler Stretch	4 Plié Slide	_____	_____ sec.
	5 Reverse Lunge	_____	_____ sec.
Flat Back Hamstring (toe flexed)	6 Outer Thigh	_____	_____ sec.
	7 Chest Press	_____	_____ sec.
Double Knee to Chest	8 Bent-Over Row	_____	_____ sec.
Side Quad Stretch	9 Upright Row	_____	_____ sec.
	10 Overhead Press	_____	_____ sec.
Child Stretch	11 Biceps Curl	_____	_____ sec.
Calf Stretch	12 Triceps Extension	_____	_____ sec.
	13 Abdominal Crunch	_____	_____ sec.
	14 Side Crunch	_____	_____ sec.
	15 Reverse Crunch	_____	_____ sec.
	16 Prone Hyperextension #2	_____	_____ sec.

10 Daily Logs:

Weeks Eight
Through Ten

PEAK WEEKS: WEEK EIGHT, DAY ONE   DATE: _____

DAILY NOTICE: Time to push it to the top.

Congratulations! You have made it through seven weeks of the Peak 10 program. At this point the summit is starting to come into view. By completing all the workouts and maintaining a well-balanced eating plan, you should be feeling your oats, or at least eating them. You should be real proud of yourself for sticking to what some think is impossible. You have worked hard and made the time to better yourself and your life. Hopefully you are sharing your newfound knowledge with your friends and loved ones, so that they too will embrace a healthier life.

Take a look at the rest of the week ahead, set your schedule, and organize your time. Balance your efforts equally between all areas of the program. Remember that you are an individual and might need to work on one area of the program more than another. Some people have to work hard to modify their diets, whereas others need to boost endurance. Work to identify and strengthen your weaknesses. In the closing weeks of the program review all the past weeks' notes to pinpoint where you need to focus. This

---

is a study of your physical life. Peak 10 will allow you to achieve more than just a passing grade.

You will be spending more time in the core segment of the fat burner. Don't forget to stretch before and after each workout. As the intensity increases, you will need more water as you exercise. Make sure to have plenty available.

Aerobic Activity	Activity	Warm-up	Core	Cool-down
Fat Burner/Warm-up		10 min.	45 min.	5 min.

Pre/Post Workout Stretch
Neck Stretch
Chest/Biceps
Shoulder/Upper Back
Modified Hurdler Stretch
Flat Back Hamstring (toe flexed)
Double Knee to Chest
Side Quad Stretch
Child Stretch
Calf Stretch

DAILY NOTICE: Rest and stretch if needed.

I encourage you to try to permanently modify your eating habits to be closer to the ones that you've had during this program. If you have a family or roommates, it wouldn't hurt them to follow a more healthful eating plan also. As a bonus, this will make it easier for you to stick with it. Eat lean, be lean.

PEAK WEEKS: WEEK EIGHT, DAY THREE DATE: _____

DAILY NOTICE: The longer you go, the more you will burn.

You will be spending more time in the core segment of the fat burner. Don't forget to stretch before and after each workout. Make sure to drink plenty of water before, during, and after exercise.

Throw on a pot of beans for some beans and rice tonight. All this extra work usually requires some "stick to your ribs" kind of food. But it doesn't have to be high in fat and calories!

AEROBIC ACTIVITY	ACTIVITY	WARM-UP	CORE	COOL-DOWN
Fat Burner/Warm-up		10 min.	45 min.	5 min.

PRE/POST WORKOUT STRETCH
Neck Stretch
Chest/Biceps
Shoulder/Upper Back
Modified Hurdler Stretch
Flat Back Hamstring (toe flexed)
Double Knee to Chest
Side Quad Stretch
Child Stretch
Calf Stretch

PEAK WEEKS: WEEK EIGHT, DAY FOUR   DATE: _____

DAILY NOTICE: Work those abs!

Start off with a 25-minute cardio-conditioning workout. After your cardio it's just abs today. Remember to stay focused when training your abdominals and lower back and always keep your lower back supported. As always, work to failure during each exercise. "Failure" means that you can't possibly do another rep. You should be familiar with that sensation by now and be comfortable pushing for it. How does your number of repetitions compare to the last time you did abs? Push out a few more this time.

Cut up some luscious fruit to snack on for the next couple of days. Try some apples, peaches, pears, and bananas with fresh lemon squeezed on top. Enjoy it!

Aerobic Activity	Activity	Warm-up	Core	Cool-down
Cardio Conditioning		5 min.	15 min.	5 min.

Pre/Post Workout Stretch	Hot Spots—Just Abs	Reps	Recovery
Neck Stretch	1 Abdominal Crunch	_____	_____ sec.
Chest/Biceps	2 Side Crunch	_____	_____ sec.
Shoulder/Upper Back	3 Reverse Crunch	_____	_____ sec.
Modified Hurdler Stretch	4 Prone Hyperextension #2	_____	_____ sec.
Flat Back Hamstring (toe flexed)			
Double Knee to Chest			
Side Quad Stretch			
Child Stretch			
Calf Stretch			

PEAK WEEKS: WEEK EIGHT, DAY FIVE   DATE: _____

DAILY NOTICE: Rest and stretch if needed.

If you need to do some grocery shopping, take the time to compare the labels of potato chips vs. pretzels, or donuts vs. toast and jam. Make the Peak 10 choice.

PEAK WEEKS: WEEK EIGHT, DAY SIX   DATE: _____

DAILY NOTICE: Take down the core for a light fat burner.

Warm up slow and keep a moderate pace for the core. Don't forget to cool down and stretch it out. It's a light day so be sure to modify your food intake accordingly. You won't need to eat as much as on those more intense workout days.

Remember that if you don't eat it, you won't have to burn it off later.

AEROBIC ACTIVITY	ACTIVITY	WARM-UP	CORE	COOL-DOWN
Fat Burner/Warm-up		10 min.	30 min.	5 min.

PRE/POST WORKOUT STRETCH
Neck Stretch
Chest/Biceps
Shoulder/Upper Back
Modified Hurdler Stretch
Flat Back Hamstring (toe flexed)
Double Knee to Chest
Side Quad Stretch
Child Stretch
Calf Stretch

DAILY NOTICE: You are ready to take on the Peak Circuit.

In the Peak Circuit you will move through the string of exercises with little or no rest. You will notice that in most cases you will perform lower body exercise and move immediately to an upper body activity.

Like the other workout circuits, it is best to lay out the exercises ahead of time. Know where to use your props for the workout (a chair, a pillow, weights, etc.) and clear the area so it is safe from obstacles. Refer back to the photos and descriptions in chapter 6 should you need assistance.

As you move through these last few weeks of the program, you will come to appreciate how fit you have become. Always remember that it's you against you. Compete with yourself and shoot for one rep more than last time.

When you challenge yourself, you will improve.

AEROBIC ACTIVITY	ACTIVITY	WARM-UP	CORE	COOL-DOWN
Cardio Conditioning		5 min.	10 min.	2 min.

PRE/POST WORKOUT STRETCH	TONING EXERCISES	REPS	RECOVERY
Neck Stretch	1 Lunge	_____	_____ sec.
Chest/Biceps	2 Chest Press	_____	_____ sec.
Shoulder/Upper Back	3 Leg Extension	_____	_____ sec.
Modified Hurdler Stretch	4 Bent-Over Row	_____	_____ sec.
Flat Back Hamstring (toe flexed)	5 Leg Curl	_____	_____ sec.
	6 Upright Row	_____	_____ sec.
Double Knee to Chest	7 Plié Slide	_____	_____ sec.
Side Quad Stretch	8 Overhead Press	_____	_____ sec.
Child Stretch	9 Reverse Lunge	_____	_____ sec.
Calf Stretch	10 Biceps Curl	_____	_____ sec.
	11 Outer Thigh	_____	_____ sec.
	12 Triceps Dip	_____	_____ sec.
	13 Abdominal Crunch	_____	_____ sec.
	14 Side Crunch	_____	_____ sec.
	15 Reverse Crunch	_____	_____ sec.
	16 Prone Hyperextension #2	_____	_____ sec.

DAILY NOTICE: Measure today!

This is the next to the last measurement day for you. As always, measure yourself before you exercise and chart your numbers next to the previous ones in the appendix. Take a look at your numbers. I hope that you're really pleased with your progress. If you still have more change to make, then get on it. These are your last two weeks to turn it up and get the most out of the program. There is no room for slacking here. Follow all details to a T and you'll see the results that you want.

Don't forget to stick to the eating plan. This is the missing link if you want better results. You are the only one who knows what you're doing and what you *should* be doing. This might be a great time to start a two-week Dietary Recall before the end of the program. Write down everything and you'll see where you need improvement. Go for it.

AEROBIC ACTIVITY	ACTIVITY	WARM-UP	CORE	COOL-DOWN
Fat Burner/Warm-up		10 min.	30 min.	5 min.

PRE/POST WORKOUT STRETCH
Neck Stretch
Chest/Biceps
Shoulder/Upper Back
Modified Hurdler Stretch
Flat Back Hamstring (toe flexed)
Double Knee to Chest
Side Quad Stretch
Child Stretch
Calf Stretch

DAILY NOTICE: Warm up with light cardio for the Peak Circuit.

Let's get started with a quick 14-minute warm-up to your strength-training routine. I don't want you to wear yourself out on the cardio segment; let's save all the juice for the training.

I want you to really train hard today. Before you start your workout, have your previous numbers in front of you. You should see improvements across the board. Compete against yourself by beating your own numbers. Set a goal for yourself and drive through to the end.

Reward your hard work with plenty of water, a nice piece of grilled fish, all the veggies you can eat. Take a bite from someone else's dessert to squelch that sweet tooth. Keep climbing.

AEROBIC ACTIVITY	ACTIVITY	WARM-UP	CORE	COOL-DOWN
Cardio Conditioning		3 min.	8 min.	3 min.

PRE/POST WORKOUT STRETCH	TONING EXERCISES	REPS	RECOVERY
Neck Stretch	1 Lunge	_____	_____ sec.
Chest/Biceps	2 Chest Press	_____	_____ sec.
Shoulder/Upper Back	3 Leg Extension	_____	_____ sec.
Modified Hurdler Stretch	4 Bent-Over Row	_____	_____ sec.
	5 Leg Curl	_____	_____ sec.
Flat Back Hamstring (toe flexed)	6 Upright Row	_____	_____ sec.
	7 Plié Slide	_____	_____ sec.
Double Knee to Chest	8 Overhead Press	_____	_____ sec.
Side Quad Stretch	9 Reverse Lunge	_____	_____ sec.
Child Stretch	10 Biceps Curl	_____	_____ sec.
Calf Stretch	11 Outer Thigh	_____	_____ sec.
	12 Triceps Dip	_____	_____ sec.
	13 Abdominal Crunch	_____	_____ sec.
	14 Side Crunch	_____	_____ sec.
	15 Reverse Crunch	_____	_____ sec.
	16 Prone Hyperextension #2	_____	_____ sec.

PEAK WEEKS: WEEK NINE, DAY THREE   DATE: _____

DAILY NOTICE: Rest and stretch if needed.

You worked really hard yesterday, so give your muscles a day off. You might need an extra good stretch today if your muscles are sore. See if you can work in a back rub. You deserve it.

PEAK WEEKS: WEEK NINE, DAY FOUR   DATE: _____

DAILY NOTICE: Aim to shorten your training time.

By now you should be able to fly through these exercises without even looking at the book. You know your proper form and you're sticking to it. And pushing yourself to muscular failure has become fun for you. The workout that used to take you an hour should take you less and less time now. Maybe you're down to 40 minutes top to bottom. That's great, and exactly what you should be doing. You can now accomplish a great workout in half the time, so you have time left over for other things.

Keep up the healthful eating habits. Most of my clients get into good "ruts" when it comes to eating. You should have your favorite recipes and snacks, you should know the best times of day for you to eat for high energy and good digestion, you should have your favorite store to find the best fresh fruits and veggies, and you should be drinking tons of water and "keeping it clear."

AEROBIC ACTIVITY	ACTIVITY	WARM-UP	CORE	COOL-DOWN
Cardio Conditioning		3 min.	8 min.	3 min.

PRE/POST WORKOUT STRETCH	TONING EXERCISES	REPS	RECOVERY
Neck Stretch	1 Lunge	————	———— sec.
Chest/Biceps	2 Chest Press	————	———— sec.
Shoulder/Upper Back	3 Leg Extension	————	———— sec.
Modified Hurdler Stretch	4 Bent-Over Row	————	———— sec.
	5 Leg Curl	————	———— sec.
Flat Back Hamstring (toe flexed)	6 Upright Row	————	———— sec.
Double Knee to Chest	7 Plié Slide	————	———— sec.
Side Quad Stretch	8 Overhead Press	————	———— sec.
Child Stretch	9 Reverse Lunge	————	———— sec.
Calf Stretch	10 Biceps Curl	————	———— sec.
	11 Outer Thigh	————	———— sec.
	12 Triceps Dip	————	———— sec.
	13 Abdominal Crunch	————	———— sec.
	14 Side Crunch	————	———— sec.
	15 Reverse Crunch	————	———— sec.
	16 Prone Hyperextension #2	————	———— sec.

DAILY NOTICE: Maintain the intensity in the core.

Take your favorite tunes with you today for extra motivation. Stay strong throughout the workout. Maybe it's time to add something a little different. Try bike riding or in-line skating alternated with power walking. Just be sure to keep your heart rate up there throughout the 45-minute core of your workout.

Are you limiting your salt intake? If you find that you're retaining water, or not losing body fat as fast as you think you should be, try cutting more salt out of your diet while increasing your water intake. Maybe your body is just hanging on to some extra fluids. Watch for high sodium in soups, soy sauce, prepared foods, pretzels, etc.

AEROBIC ACTIVITY	ACTIVITY	WARM-UP	CORE	COOL-DOWN
Fat Burner/Warm-up		10 min.	45 min.	5 min.

PRE/POST WORKOUT STRETCH
Neck Stretch
Chest/Biceps
Shoulder/Upper Back
Modified Hurdler Stretch
Flat Back Hamstring (toe flexed)
Double Knee to Chest
Side Quad Stretch
Child Stretch
Calf Stretch

DAILY NOTICE: Finish the week strong.

This is your last training day of week nine. Let's get the most out of it. We're going to start out with a good warm-up to lower your risk of injury. Then we're going to take you through a Peak Circuit. Remember, that means that you're shooting for little or no rest between sets, but be sure to keep good form throughout. Have some water on hand—you might need it. Push through your sets, beating your last numbers. This is the best way to see yourself getting stronger. Enjoy the sweet satisfaction of being successful.

AEROBIC ACTIVITY	ACTIVITY	WARM-UP	CORE	COOL-DOWN
Cardio Conditioning		3 min.	8 min.	3 min.

PRE/POST WORKOUT STRETCH	TONING EXERCISES	REPS	RECOVERY
Neck Stretch	1 Lunge	_____	_____ sec.
Chest/Biceps	2 Chest Press	_____	_____ sec.
Shoulder/Upper Back	3 Leg Extension	_____	_____ sec.
Modified Hurdler Stretch	4 Bent-Over Row	_____	_____ sec.
Flat Back Hamstring (toe flexed)	5 Leg Curl	_____	_____ sec.
	6 Upright Row	_____	_____ sec.
Double Knee to Chest	7 Plié Slide	_____	_____ sec.
Side Quad Stretch	8 Overhead Press	_____	_____ sec.
Child Stretch	9 Reverse Lunge	_____	_____ sec.
Calf Stretch	10 Biceps Curl	_____	_____ sec.
	11 Outer Thigh	_____	_____ sec.
	12 Triceps Dip	_____	_____ sec.
	13 Abdominal Crunch	_____	_____ sec.
	14 Side Crunch	_____	_____ sec.
	15 Reverse Crunch	_____	_____ sec.
	16 Prone Hyperextension #2	_____	_____ sec.

DAILY NOTICE: Rest and stretch if needed.

Take the day to savor your accomplishments. Tomorrow you will start the tenth and final week of your program. You can see the peak of the mountain in the distance, and you're almost there.

PEAK WEEKS: WEEK TEN, DAY ONE

DAILY NOTICE: Burn fat, strengthen and tone your abs.

Yippee! You've reached the tenth week of your ten-week program. Most of this should be automatic for you now. Today we will do an hour of cardio and then finish up with an intense ab workout. Really push yourself on those abs. I know you can add another 5 reps to each exercise.

In honor of ab day, I want you to plan your next three days of meals, including two or three servings per day of fruit and veggies. All this exercise requires good nutrition.

AEROBIC ACTIVITY	ACTIVITY	WARM-UP	CORE	COOL-DOWN
Fat Burner/Warm-up		10 min.	45 min.	5 min.

PRE/POST WORKOUT STRETCH	HOT SPOTS—JUST ABS	REPS	RECOVERY
Neck Stretch	1 Abdominal Crunch	_____	_____ sec.
Chest/Biceps	2 Side Crunch	_____	_____ sec.
Shoulder/Upper Back	3 Reverse Crunch	_____	_____ sec.
Modified Hurdler Stretch	4 Prone Hyperextension #2	_____	_____ sec.
Flat Back Hamstring (toe flexed)			
Double Knee to Chest			
Side Quad Stretch			
Child Stretch			
Calf Stretch			

PEAK WEEKS: WEEK TEN, DAY TWO   DATE: _____

DAILY NOTICE: Rest and stretch if needed.

Take this time to go through the kitchen cupboards and fridge again. Sometimes a little junk food sneaks in from time to time. Now's the time to clear it out and move on in a positive vein. I know that following each holiday, there are a few "gifts" that can tend to derail my efforts, so nip that in the bud and get rid of it now! Don't hesitate giving it away or throwing it out.

PEAK WEEKS: WEEK TEN, DAY THREE   DATE: _____

DAILY NOTICE: Warm up with light cardio for the Peak Circuit.

Warm up and work your core in the high end of your Target Training Zone. Really push it to condition your heart. Cool down and begin your Peak Circuit. Watch your form throughout your routine. Remember that when you start to break form, you're beginning to reach failure. You must correct your form and push through the last rep.

Wear clothing that will allow you to see your muscles working. As tacky as it sounds, a tank top or crop top is usually the best thing to wear to see those muscles. Take pride in how firm and toned your body looks. Start looking at where you want to further sculpt and define.

Remember that your diet plays a large role in this too. Stay strict with yourself. A little here and a little there will quickly add up to extra ripples in the wrong places. Pay close attention to everything you put into your body.

Aerobic Activity	Activity	Warm-up	Core	Cool-down
Cardio Conditioning		3 min.	8 min.	3 min.

Pre/Post Workout Stretch	Toning Exercises	Reps	Recovery
Neck Stretch	1 Lunge	_____	_____ sec.
Chest/Biceps	2 Chest Press	_____	_____ sec.
Shoulder/Upper Back	3 Leg Extension	_____	_____ sec.
Modified Hurdler Stretch	4 Bent-Over Row	_____	_____ sec.
Flat Back Hamstring (toe flexed)	5 Leg Curl	_____	_____ sec.
	6 Upright Row	_____	_____ sec.
Double Knee to Chest	7 Plié Slide	_____	_____ sec.
Side Quad Stretch	8 Overhead Press	_____	_____ sec.
Child Stretch	9 Reverse Lunge	_____	_____ sec.
Calf Stretch	10 Biceps Curl	_____	_____ sec.
	11 Outer Thigh	_____	_____ sec.
	12 Triceps Dip	_____	_____ sec.
	13 Abdominal Crunch	_____	_____ sec.
	14 Side Crunch	_____	_____ sec.
	15 Reverse Crunch	_____	_____ sec.
	16 Prone Hyperextension #2	_____	_____ sec.

DAILY NOTICE: Get comfortable in the core.

This is your last big cardio day. Take it outside and make it special. Try something a little more intense. Walk, run, or bike a little further than usual in the same amount of time. Savor the endorphin rush that you get from working in your fat-burning zone. Remember always to use the proper safety equipment for whatever activity you plan to do.

Have dinner with a friend to celebrate the last week of your Peak 10 program. As always, make it healthful.

AEROBIC ACTIVITY	ACTIVITY	WARM-UP	CORE	COOL-DOWN
Fat Burner/Warm-up		10 min.	45 min.	5 min.

PRE/POST WORKOUT STRETCH

Neck Stretch

Chest/Biceps

Shoulder/Upper Back

Modified Hurdler Stretch

Flat Back Hamstring (toe flexed)

Double Knee to Chest

Side Quad Stretch

Child Stretch

Calf Stretch

DAILY NOTICE: Light warm-up and stretch.

An 18-minute cardio warm-up and a really good stretch will help cool you down from the last few weeks of intense training. Remember that this routine is always great, even after you've finished the program, to relax and refresh you. Be sure to drink lots of water in the next couple of days to prevent bloating on your final measuring day. You've done a terrific job so far. You should be very proud of yourself. You've followed these routines with enough consistency to instill some permanent change in your habits. The rest is downhill. It should be easy to continue exercising and eating right. You will feel as though something is wrong when you *don't* exercise or if you eat junky food. Stick with those healthful patterns.

AEROBIC ACTIVITY	ACTIVITY	WARM-UP	CORE	COOL-DOWN
Fat Burner/Warm-up		5 min.	10 min.	3 min.

PRE/POST WORKOUT STRETCH
Neck Stretch
Chest/Biceps
Shoulder/Upper Back
Modified Hurdler Stretch
Flat Back Hamstring (toe flexed)
Double Knee to Chest
Side Quad Stretch
Child Stretch
Calf Stretch

DAILY NOTICE: Finish the program strong.

This is your last training day on the program. You've stuck with it to the end and have done a great job. You are seeing positive changes in your body, inside and out. You have taken control of the program and made it work for you. Now you know that you can succeed in any aspect of your life. And the positive changes that you see don't have to be the end of your improvements. You can continue to improve your body from here forward. You might not progress with the same intensity, but the whole point is that we are all works in progress, and we all have plenty of room for improvement no matter what we look like.

Continue to plan out your meals in advance. If you save the fatty and sugary foods for limited occasions and small quantities, then you don't have to swear off them for life. You can go out and feel comfortable having an occasional glass of wine, or a bite of cake, or a little olive oil, as long as you don't do them all at once. Now power through your final workout and finish the program strong.

Aerobic Activity	Activity	Warm-up	Core	Cool-down
Cardio Conditioning		3 min.	8 min.	3 min.

Pre/Post Workout Stretch	Toning Exercises	Reps	Recovery
Neck Stretch	1 Lunge	_____	_____ sec.
Chest/Biceps	2 Chest Press	_____	_____ sec.
Shoulder/Upper Back	3 Leg Extension	_____	_____ sec.
Modified Hurdler Stretch	4 Bent-Over Row	_____	_____ sec.
Flat Back Hamstring (toe flexed)	5 Leg Curl	_____	_____ sec.
	6 Upright Row	_____	_____ sec.
Double Knee to Chest	7 Plié Slide	_____	_____ sec.
Side Quad Stretch	8 Overhead Press	_____	_____ sec.
Child Stretch	9 Reverse Lunge	_____	_____ sec.
Calf Stretch	10 Biceps Curl	_____	_____ sec.
	11 Outer Thigh	_____	_____ sec.
	12 Triceps Dip	_____	_____ sec.
	13 Abdominal Crunch	_____	_____ sec.
	14 Side Crunch	_____	_____ sec.
	15 Reverse Crunch	_____	_____ sec.
	16 Prone Hyperextension #2	_____	_____ sec.

DAILY NOTICE: Congratulations, you did it!!!

At long last. You might feel like this has been a long time coming. But you're finally at the top of the mountain. You are an official graduate of the Peak 10 program. Now it is time for you to take final measurements and the program-ending pictures from your miraculous vantage point. You will take your "after" pictures today. Now you will be able to really see how your body has changed. Look at all the great work that you've done to look and feel your very best.

Now take your final set of measurements and pat yourself on the back. Better yet, treat yourself to something special. You deserve it.

Afterword

Reaching the Top and Enjoying the View

As I've stressed throughout the book, Peak 10 was designed to help you change your current pattern of living. The whole concept of the Peak 10 program is to instill a lifelong pattern of health and fitness. In making the climb, step by step, you have discovered your body's hidden abilities to succeed regardless of the challenges. You have reached new limits that have given you a whole new view on life. You are stronger, you are leaner, and you are proud.

You made the commitment that has allowed you to experience an incredible transformation. To control your body, and to have more than just an opinion on the condition of your health, is power. In taking on this program you have taken yourself on—and won. Whether you've met your goals or not, I know at least you've looked upward to a point of higher health and fitness. Understanding what it takes to be your best is all you need. Learning the valuable lessons from a wrong turn or two is also part of the equation. The equation is a simple one. Learn and practice, learn and practice, learn and practice—it will assure improvement every time.

Capture the Moment

At the end of any climb you would take a photo to remember the accomplishment. Let's reenact the photo session you took at the beginning of the program. You should have also taken your end-of-program measurements. Tally up the total inches gained or lost and see how you did. Both the photos and the measurements are great trophies for all the time and effort that you have put into the program.

Time to ask some questions. How did you do with your goals? Did you reduce your body fat? Are you stronger and leaner? Do you have greater endurance? These are all very important questions. They will be able to provide you with more information. If you have made great strides in the program, once again, super job! If you fell short in specific areas, reevaluate. Were you honest with yourself? Did you make a real effort to change? Did you follow the program without resistance? Did you let others influence your commitment? This program was designed to instill change. Reaching your goals is an important part of this program but not its main objective. If you continue to walk out your front door with the intention of increasing your heart rate, or find yourself on your treadmill at a time when you would normally be kicking back a cocktail or two, *you have made change,* positive change. And it is changes like these that will bring about physical improvements over time. It is just a matter of making health-provoking choices a normal part of your everyday life.

Above the Clouds

"The hard thing was ending it," explains Martha McCully. "My body felt so clean. I had to find a balance and not be obsessive because Peak 10 is a lifestyle, not a diet. I kept telling myself that."

"I've altered the way I live. I educated myself. I feel better about myself," says Carol Lynde. "I learned my capabilities through this program. I learned how strong I am. I feel strong, like I'm going in the right direction in life. I have my head on straight."

Carol says that she always reminds herself how great she felt when she successfully completed Peak 10. Remembering, reminding, and the reinforcement of the feelings of accomplishment and achievement are what you need to do. Now that the program is behind you, you need to know what to do. You have a world of knowledge and over seventy-five hours of practical experience, not to mention the bod to show for all your efforts. You will only get better if you continue to understand the balance that you have created between you and the world around you.

FIND THE TIME TO FIT IT ALL IN

There are 168 hours in each week. That's 24 hours in each day, seven days in each week. *168 hours!* That's a lot of time when you add it up and look at the big picture. I know from my own life, with my wife, Sally, and my one-year-old son, T. Rex (that's short for Tyler Rex), along with our own business and never-ending special projects, that even with all those hours it's sometimes hard to fit it all in. This is why it's crucially important to try to *live* fitness. You wake up in the morning, have a supercharged breakfast, and plan out your day. Incorporate your workout with your children or parents. Make it a social event. Talk about it at the dinner table. It makes better conversation than what's in the newspapers these days, and it also will help you gain the support of others. If being fit and working out become a normal part of your life, looking great and feeling great will too.

TRAINING TIPS TO MAINTAIN OR IMPROVE YOUR BODY

Weight-train twice a week with your Peak Circuit.
Incorporate the Hot Spots exercises that you need.
Do the cardiovascular and fat-burning exercises two or three times a week.
Make the time for it and it will keep you in the shape you're enjoying
   today.

SHOULD YOU DO ANOTHER PEAK 10?

Peak 10 wasn't designed to be done at the same level of intensity for the rest of your life. However, the components are each a reasonable part of a healthy lifestyle. By continuing to practice these components in moderation, including aerobic training, strength training, and of course a healthful, low-fat, high-fiber diet, you will continue to become your very best. Remember, your health and fitness are what they are because of what you do.

If you want to continue to improve your body, continue to lead a life full of fitness, fun, and healthful eating. If you want to move faster, you know just how to "turn it up." I've given you all the tools that you need to continue climbing. The only difference is, now *you* are the guide leading this expedition. And you know exactly what to do, because you've come to know yourself better through this experience. Welcome to your new life.

KITTY'S STORY

I went through breast cancer, chemotherapy, and finally surgery, which meant taking a lot of medication that made me fat and puffy. I couldn't get my weight down even though I was eating nothing. I ate a lot of fat-free junk and pretzels, but I wasn't nourished. And I couldn't get my activity level high enough to burn any calories. I needed something to jump start a change in my situation. After you go through something like surgery or pregnancy you have a perfect excuse to be fat. I could be 50 pounds overweight for the rest of my life and everyone would understand, but why should I do that to myself? I was completely sure Peak 10 was a healthy way to get back in shape.

Kitty Age: 39 Height: 5'2"	*Start*	*Finish*
MEASUREMENTS		
Neck	13.25	11.75
Shoulders	37.75	37
Chest	35.25	34.5
Waist	29.5	27.5
Hips	35.75	35
Rt. Thigh	22	19.75
Rt. Calf	13.75	13
Rt. Upper Arm	11.5	10.25
Rt. Forearm	9.5	9
Weight	129	118
% Fat	28/29.8	25.1/24.5
TOTAL INCHES	208.25	197.75
Inches lost: 10.50		

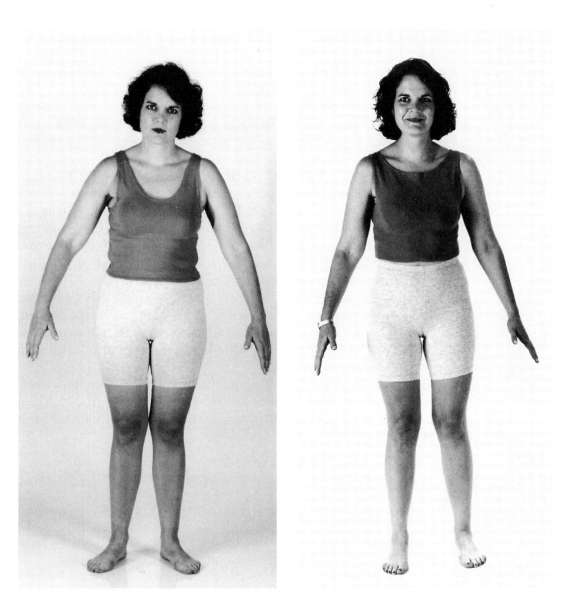

I called the doctors and they had some concern because of reconstructive surgery, since the prosthetic is under the muscle, but any type of exercise you do is good. It was more than good—they thought it was fabulous.

I had always wondered if I could do it like the movie stars do it—go away and work out and eat right every day and then look good. Peak 10 seemed like the next best thing to spending a lot of money at a spa for six months.

I went out for runs before or after work and took really long walks on the weekends. Exercise is a wonderful time to meditate. I took a radio with me and started listening to National Public Radio or a country station or salsa station. I'd flip back and forth—it was a blast. Walking or running is also a great time to get peace and quiet and do mental problem-solving.

I was really good about diet. After I got started I thought I'd crave chocolate and all kinds of stuff, but I really didn't. I went months without chocolate and I didn't care. I never felt the urge to binge. I actually ate more on Peak 10—more fresh vegetables and salads. I started eating salads with vinegar. For dinner I'd have pasta or vegetables. It wasn't tough. I also read nutrition labels carefully because a lot of products present themselves as good for you when they are not.

Eventually, I lost 20 pounds. I threw out all my old clothes and had everything fitted. At the end, I looked really good. Everybody said, "Wow, look at you." I got to where I hadn't been in years. I bought a size four pants, which I hadn't bought since before I was married, although most everything else is a size six.

Chris straightened out my eating plan and taught me the right exercises to do. For me Peak 10 was an opportunity to get into the best physical shape possible. You really can do it yourself and still have your regular life.

Appendix I

Taking Measurements

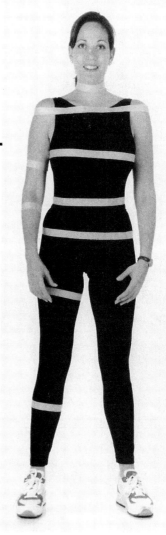

PEAK 10 PROGRESS CHART

Name: _____

Age: _____

	Before	Week 2	Week 4	Week 6	Week 8	Week 10
Date:						
Time:						
MEASUREMENTS (inches)						
Neck						
Shoulders						
Chest						
Waist						
Hips						
Rt. Thigh						
Rt. Calf						
Rt. Upper Arm						
Rt. Forearm						
TOTAL INCHES						
Weight						
%Fat						
Height						

Appendix II

Dietary Recall

DIETARY RECALL

Day 1	Breakfast	Mid-morning	Lunch	Mid-afternoon	Dinner	PM Snack
Time						
Food/ Beverage						
Where are you?						
Who is with you?						
What are you doing?						
How do you feel?						

Notes:

Dietary Recall (CONTINUED)

Day 2	Breakfast	Mid-morning	Lunch	Mid-afternoon	Dinner	PM Snack
Time						
Food/ Beverage						
Where are you?						
Who is with you?						
What are you doing?						
How do you feel?						
Notes:						

DIETARY RECALL (CONTINUED)

Day 3	Breakfast	Mid-morning	Lunch	Mid-afternoon	Dinner	PM Snack
Time						
Food/ Beverage						
Where are you?						
Who is with you?						
What are you doing?						
How do you feel?						
Notes:						

Dietary Recall (CONTINUED)

Day 4	Breakfast	Mid-morning	Lunch	Mid-afternoon	Dinner	PM Snack
Time						
Food/ Beverage						
Where are you?						
Who is with you?						
What are you doing?						
How do you feel?						
Notes:						

DIETARY RECALL (CONTINUED)

Day 5	Breakfast	Mid-morning	Lunch	Mid-afternoon	Dinner	PM Snack
Time						
Food/ Beverage						
Where are you?						
Who is with you?						
What are you doing?						
How do you feel?						

Notes:

DIETARY RECALL (CONTINUED)

Day 6	Breakfast	Mid-morning	Lunch	Mid-afternoon	Dinner	PM Snack
Time						
Food/ Beverage						
Where are you?						
Who is with you?						
What are you doing?						
How do you feel?						
Notes:						

DIETARY RECALL (CONTINUED)

Day 7	Breakfast	Mid-morning	Lunch	Mid-afternoon	Dinner	PM Snack
Time						
Food/ Beverage						
Where are you?						
Who is with you?						
What are you doing?						
How do you feel?						

Notes:

Now Available on Home Video:
Chris Imbo's Peak 10 Fitness Program

A perfect complement to the full PEAK 10 program detailed in the book, Chris Imbo's PEAK 10 videos allow you to use your VCR to help keep you even more motivated throughout the program and to get into the best shape of your life!

Have Chris and his exercise partner supermodel Frederique lead you through a challenging upper and lower body exercise routine which can easily be exchanged for the book's toning segments. Each video also includes "world class" aerobics sessions led by renowned aerobics instructor Kacy Duke, which are a great rainy day alternative to your regular outdoor aerobic work.

Order today and you will receive:

> 1. PEAK 10 Volume One, featuring Abs and Upper Body Sculpting plus Fat Burning Aerobics

and

> 2. PEAK 10 Volume Two, featuring Lower Body Sculpting plus Energy Building Aerobics.

Each video includes 75 minutes of Chris's highly acclaimed exercises.

Both videos are available to buyers of Chris Imbo's PEAK 10 book for a special price of $19.95 (plus $4.95 shipping and handling). Call 1-800-321-4420. Visa or MasterCard accepted, or send check or money order to PEAk 10 Fitness, P.O. Box 9386, Canoga Park, CA 91309. California and Connecticut residents please add sales tax.